Testbank to Accompany

FUNDAMENTALS OF
NURSING
THE ART AND SCIENCE OF NURSING CARE

D1552137

Testbank to Accompany

FUNDAMENTALS OF
NURSING
THE ART AND SCIENCE OF NURSING CARE

Third Edition

PREPARED BY

Diane Billings, RN, FAAN, EdD
Professor of Nursing
Assistant Dean of Learning Resources
Indiana University
School of Nursing
Indianapolis, Indiana

Karen L. Cobb, RN, EdD
Assistant Professor of Nursing
Indiana University
School of Nursing
Indianapolis, Indiana

Teresa M. Dobrzykowski, RN, MSN
Lecturer, Indiana University
School of Nursing
South Bend, Indiana

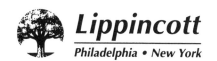
Lippincott
Philadelphia • New York

Acquisition Editor: Mary Gyetvan
Assistant Editor: Susan Keneally
Ancillary Editor: Doris S. Wray
Senior Production Manager: Janet Greenwood
Production Services: Berliner Inc.
Printer/Binder: Courier Kendallville

Third Edition

ISBN: 0-397-55764-7

Care has been taken to confirm the accuracy of the information presented and to describe generally accepted practices. However, the authors, editors, and publisher are not responsible for errors or omissions or for any consequences from application of the information in this book and make no warranty, express or implied, with respect to the contents of the publication.

The authors, editors, and publisher have exerted every effort to ensure that drug selection and dosage set forth in this text are in accordance with current recommendations and practice at the time of publication. However, in view of ongoing research, changes in government regulations, and the constant flow of information relating to drug therapy and drug reactions, the reader is urged to check the package insert for each drug for any change in indications and dosages and for added warnings and precautions. This is particularly important when the recommended agent is a new or infrequently employed drug.

Some drugs and medical devices presented in this publication have Food and Drug Administration (FDA) clearance for limited use in restricted research settings. It is the responsibility of the health care provider to ascertain the FDA status of each drug or device planned for use in their clinical practice.

9 8 7 6 5 4 3 2 1

Introduction

The testbank for Taylor's *Fundamentals of Nursing: The Art and Science of Nursing Care,* 3rd edition consists of approximately 1000 multiple-choice questions. All questions are coded for the level of difficulty and are cross-referenced to the page where the topic is discussed and the correct answer can be found.

Accompanying each item in this testbank is a set of item descriptors printed below each question. The descriptors contain basic infomation about an item and are used to determine which items you would like to include on a test. Thus, you will be able to sort questions based on these criteria. The following key explains the descriptors used in this testbank.

Example:

< 1 >   1. A client is scheduled to have surgery on his feet in an ambulatory surgery facility. Before the surgery is performed, the nurse should determine if the client
< 2 >   *A. has had appropriate screening tests.
             B. has assistance from a family member at home.
             C. needs a bath or shower with betadine soap.
             D. should be admitted to the hospital following surgery.
< 3 >   Reference: p. 194

Descriptors: < 4 > 12   < 5 > 04   < 6 > Application
               < 7 > 2   < 8 > Moderate

Key:

< 1 >   Question number
< 2 >   Correct answer
< 3 >   Referenced page number (from textbook)
< 4 >   Chapter number
< 5 >   Chapter objective
< 6 >   Cognitive type (application, factual, interpretive)
< 7 >   Step of the Nursing Process
        1 = No Process
        2 = Assessment
        3 = Analysis/Diagnosis
        4 = Planning
        5 = Implementation
        6 = Evaluation
< 8 >   Difficulty Level (easy, moderate, difficult)

All questions in this testbank are multiple choice.

Contents

UNIT I: Foundations for Nursing Practice

1 Introduction to Nursing 1
2 Basic Human Needs: Individual, Family, and Community 2
3 Culture and Ethnicity.. 3
4 Promoting Wellness in Health and Illness 4
5 Theoretical Base for Nursing Practice 5
6 Values and Ethics in Nursing 6
7 Legal Implications in Nursing... 9

UNIT II: Promoting Wellness Across the Life Span

8 Developmental Concepts 13
9 Conception Through Adolescence 14
10 Early, Middle, and Older Adulthood 16

UNIT III: Community-Based Settings for Client Care

11 Community-Based Health Care 18
12 Continuity of Care 19
13 Home Health Care 20

UNIT IV: The Nursing Process

14 Introduction to Nursing Process 22
15 Essential Knowledge and Skills in Nursing 22
16 Assessing 23
17 Diagnosing 24
18 Planning 25
19 Implementing 27
20 Evaluating 27
21 Documenting, Reporting, and Conferring... 28

UNIT V: Roles Basic to Nursing Care

22 Communicator 30
23 Teacher and Counselor 31
24 Leader, Researcher, and Advocate 32

UNIT VI: Actions Basic to Nursing Care

25 Vital Signs 34
26 Health Assessment 37
27 Safety.. 41
28 Asepsis.. 43
29 Medications.. 47
30 Perioperative Nursing 54

UNIT VII: Promoting Healthy Psychosocial Responses

31 Self-Conept 61
32 Stress and Adaptation 62
33 Loss, Grief, and Death 64
34 Sensory Stimulation 66
35 Sexuality 67
36 Spirituality.. 68

UNIT VIII: Promoting Healthy Physiologic Responses

37 Hygiene 69
38 Skin Integrity 75
39 Activity 78
40 Rest and Sleep 84
41 Comfort 89
42 Nutrition 94
43 Urinary Elimination 102
44 Bowel Elimination 110
45 Oxygenation 117
46 Fluid, Electrolyte, and Acid–Base Balance 123

Testbank to Accompany

FUNDAMENTALS OF
NURSING
THE ART AND SCIENCE OF NURSING CARE

UNIT I
FOUNDATIONS FOR NURSING PRACTICE

CHAPTER 1
Introduction to Nursing

1. Which of the following actions best describes nursing as a profession and as a discipline?

   A. Historical social developments and changes
   B. Medical technological advances
   *C. Clinically based research
   D. University-based education

   Reference: p. 9

   Descriptors: 1. 01   2. 02   3. Application
   4. 1 = No Process   5. Moderate

2. Providing information about diet and exercise for a healthy diabetic client is best described as which of the following nursing activities?

   A. Promoting wellness
   *B. Preventing illness
   C. Treating disease
   D. Restoring health

   Reference: p. 10

   Descriptors: 1. 01   2. 03   3. Application
   4. 1 = No Process   5. Difficult

3. All of the following are commonly accepted roles and functions of nurses except

   A. collaborating with other health care professionals.
   B. participating in and or conduct research.
   *C. prescribing complex medical and surgical treatments.
   D. assisting clients to learn how to promote self-care activities.

   Reference: p. 10

   Descriptors: 1. 01   2. 03   3. Application
   4. 1 = No Process   5. Moderate

4. Which of the following educational levels describes the LVN (licensed visiting nurse) or LPN (licensed practical nurse)?

   *A. 1-year technical degree
   B. 2-year university degree
   C. 3-year hospital diploma
   D. 4-year university degree

   Reference: p. 12

   Descriptors: 1. 01   2. 04   3. Factual
   4. 1 = No Process   5. Easy

5. A difference between associate degree and baccalaureate degree nurses is that

   A. only associate degree nurses can provide primary client care.
   *B. baccalaureate degree nurses evaluate research for applicability to client care.
   C. associate degree nurses delegate care to other health care professionals.
   D. only baccalaureate degree nurses can utilize the nursing process for client care.

   Reference: pp. 14–15

   Descriptors: 1. 01   2. 04   3. Factual
   4. 1 = No Process   5. Easy

6. A major rationale for the development and continuation of professional nursing organizations is to

   A. provide socialization for members.
   B. regulate members' work and career activities.
   *C. set standards for nursing practice.
   D. provide relevant personal data for health care agencies.

   Reference: pp. 15–16

   Descriptors: 1. 01   2. 05   3. Interpretive
   4. 1 = No Process   5. Moderate

CHAPTER 2
Basic Human Needs: Individual, Family, and Community

1. A 2-year-old client suffering from asthma is admitted to the hospital. Which of the following is the most immediate client need for the nurse to address?

   A. Ensuring his favorite stuffed toy is at his side.
   B. Keeping the side rails up at all times.
   *C. Providing oxygen and a clear airway.
   D. Providing his favorite snack at bedtime.

   Reference: p. 22

   Descriptors: 1. 02   2. 03   3. Application
                4. 5 = Implementation 5. Difficult

2. Teaching the client about the side effects and benefits of medications coincides with which of the following levels of Maslow's hierarchy of needs?

   A. Physiologic
   *B. Safety and security
   C. Love and belonging
   D. Self-actualization

   Reference: p. 23

   Descriptors: 1. 02   2. 02   3. Interpretive
                4. 1 = No Process   5. Moderate

3. To asssist a client meet his or her self-esteem needs, the nurse should

   A. negate the client's own negative self-perceptions.
   B. compliment the client about anything to increase self-thought.
   C. determine the client's goals without his or her assistance.
   *D. accept the client's values and beliefs.

   Reference: p. 24

   Descriptors: 1. 02   2. 03   3. Application
                4. 5 = Implementation 5. Moderate

4. To promote the client's love and belonging needs, the nurse should

   *A. include significant others in the care of the client.
   B. encourage the client to set attainable goals.
   C. provide a sense of direction and hope.
   D. refer the client to group therapy.

   Reference: pp. 23–24

   Descriptors: 1. 02   2. 03   3. Application
                4. 5 = Implementation 5. Moderate

5. Traditional families may include all of the following members except

   A. biological parents.
   B. stepchildren.
   *C. grandparents.
   D. adopted children.

   Reference: pp. 24–26

   Descriptors: 1. 02   2. 01   3. Factual
                4. 1 = No Process   5. Easy

6. Which of the following societal factors is responsible for helping to change the roles of men and women in traditional families?

   A. Decreased educational opportunities for women
   B. Increased educational opportunities for men
   C. Increased economic standards of living
   *D. Increased career opportunities for women

   Reference: p. 26

   Descriptors: 1. 02   2. 04   3. Factual
                4. 1 = No Process   5. Easy

7. Serving family favorite foods and observing holidays in a prescribed manner accurately describes which family function?

   A. Physical
   B. Economic
   C. Affective
   *D. Socialization

   Reference: p. 27

   Descriptors: 1. 02   2. 04   3. Application
                4. 1 = No Process   5. Easy

8. An appropriate nursing intervention when providing family-sensitive client care to a hospitalized client is to

   A. limit the client's visitors.
   *B. encourage family to bring in favorite food and personal items.
   C. allow the client to set personal goals.
   D. provide hope and direction as needed.

   Reference: pp. 28–29

   Descriptors: 1. 02   2. 06   3. Application
                4. 5 = Implementation 5. Moderate

9. When caring for families with teenagers, the nurse should instruct the parents to

   *A. assist the teenager to balance freedom with responsibility.
   B. learn to cope with parental loss of energy.
   C. renegotiate their marital relationships.
   D. promote joint decision-making with the teenager.

   Reference: p. 28

   Descriptors: 1. 02   2. 04   3. Application
                4. 5 = Implementation 5. Moderate

10. Which of the following is considered a risk factor for family development?

A. Adequate support system readily available
B. A stable economic environment
*C. History of chronic drug abuse
D. Availability of community-based medical resources

Reference: p. 28

Descriptors: 1. 02   2. 03   3. Application
4. 2 = Assessment/3 = Analysis/Diag.
5. Moderate

CHAPTER 3
Culture and Ethnicity

1. Which of the following characteristics is a descriptor of one's race in the United States?

A. Language
B. Religion
*C. Skin color
D. Food preferences

Reference: p. 34

Descriptors: 1. 03   2. 01   3. Factual
4. 1 = No Process   5. Easy

2. The statement "When in America, you should act American" is a statement reflecting which cultural misconception?

A. Stereotyping
B. Blindness
C. Imposition
*D. Conflict

Reference: p. 35

Descriptors: 1. 03   2. 02   3. Application
4. 1 = No Process   5. Moderate

3. In caring for a Hispanic client, the nurse notes a lowering of the eyes when conversing. Culturally, this is a sign of

A. shame.
*B. deference.
C. modesty.
D. aggression.

Reference: p. 36

Descriptors: 1. 03   2. 03   3. Application
4. 2 = Assessment   5. Easy

4. When completing a cultural assessment, the nurse should consider the following:

*A. clients may prefer a health care provider of a similar cultural background.
B. knowledge of the particular language a client uses in formal conversation.
C. the type of payment plan a client will use for their health care needs.
D. talking to the client in a loud, simplified version of English will facilitate communication.

Reference: p. 36

Descriptors: 1. 03   2. 05   3. Application
4. 4 = Planning   5. Moderate

5. The most important factor to consider when caring for clients with limited income is

A. limited access to reliable transportation.
*B. basic physiologic needs left unmet.
C. limited access to health care.
D. self-actualization needs left unmet.

Reference: p. 38

Descriptors: 1. 03   2. 05   3. Factual
4. 2 = Assessment   5. Easy

6. A nurse caring for a Puerto Rican client experiencing extreme anxiety notes agitated movements resembling seizure activity. The nurse should

A. ask for a neurological consult for the abnormal behavior.
*B. stay with the client to assure behavior is culturally relevant and to ensure client safety.
C. allow the client to have privacy until the behavior returns to an acceptable level.
D. ask the client to cease the inappropriate behavior immediately.

Reference: p. 41

Descriptors: 1. 03   2. 07   3. Application
4. 5 = Implementation 5. Difficult

7. When assessing a client's pain, the nurse should

A. realize everyone's reaction to pain is similar.
B. utilize the same criteria for pain assessment for all clients.
C. encourage medically prescribed pain regimens.
*D. respect a client's individuality in pain response.

Reference: pp. 41–43

Descriptors: 1. 03   2. 05   3. Application
4. 1 = No Process   5. Moderate

8. A couple from the Philippines living in the United States is expecting their first child. In providing culturally competent care, the nurse must first

 *A. review his/her own cultural beliefs and biases.
  B. respectfully request the couple to utilize only medically approved health care providers.
  C. realize the client will have to learn their new country's accepted medical practices.
  D. study family dynamics to understand the male and female gender roles in the client's culture.

Reference: p. 44

Descriptors: 1. 03   2. 07   3. Application
             4. 5 = Implementation 5. Moderate

9. Nursing considerations when caring for African-American clients include that

  A. families are generally distant and non-supportive.
 *B. special hair and nail care may be required.
  C. fad diets are a cultural norm.
  D. clients are generally future-oriented.

Reference: p. 46

Descriptors: 1. 03   2. 07   3. Application
             4. 5 = Implementation 5. Moderate

10. When caring for a Native American family, the nurse needs to consider which of the following?

  A. The family solely consists of only the parents and children.
  B. Native Americans tend to be future-oriented.
 *C. Some Native Americans use herbs and psychologic treatment of illnesses.
  D. Health care is usually prescribed by a medicine man (shaman).

Reference: p. 49

Descriptors: 1. 03   2. 07   3. Application
             4. 1 = No Process 5. Moderate

CHAPTER 4
Promoting Wellness in Health and Illness

1. Wellness is influenced by which of the following personal factors?

  A. Community standards
 *B. Emotional needs
  C. Religious standards
  D. Professional standards

Reference: p. 53

Descriptors 1. 04   2. 02   3. Factual
             4. 1 = No Process 5. Easy

2. Illness is to disease as _____ is to heat.

  A. cold
 *B. burn
  C. anger
  D. sun

Reference: p. 53

Descriptors: 1. 04   2. 02   3. Interpretive
             4. 1 = No Process 5. Moderate

3. Appropriate nursing interventions for a client experiencing illness using Dunn's model of wellness would include

 *A. Providing holistic care as appropriate
  B. Discovering the causative agent of the disease
  C. Ascertaining the client's perception of seriousness of the disease
  D. Providing care directed solely to treat the disease

Reference: p. 54

Descriptors: 1. 04   2. 02   3. Application
             4. 5 = Implementation 5. Moderate

4. A client experiences headaches after stressful work sessions. This is an example of which of the following dimensions influencing health status?

 *A. Emotional
  B. Intellectual
  C. Physical
  D. Sociocultural

Reference: pp. 55–57

Descriptors: 1. 04   2. 03   3. Application
             4. 3 = Analysis/Diag. 5. Easy

5. A Catholic couple requests communion to be served to them and their hospitalized child prior to surgery. This is an example of which of the following needs?

  A. Environmental
  B. Physical
 *C. Spiritual
  D. Sociocultural

Reference: p. 58

Descriptors: 1. 04   2. 03   3. Application
             4. 3 = Analysis/Diag. 5. Moderate

6. An appropriate nursing diagnosis for a client experiencing dissatisfaction with their appearance is

  A. ineffective coping.
 *B. alteration in body image.
  C. grief.
  D. spiritual distress.

Reference: pp. 58–59

Descriptors: 1. 04   2. 03   3. Application
             4. 3 = Analysis/Diag. 5. Moderate

7. An example of an acute illness is

   *A. bronchitis.
   B. hypertension.
   C. asthma.
   D. arthritis.

   Reference: pp. 59–60

   Descriptors: 1. 04   2. 04   3. Factual
                4. 1 = No Process   5. Moderate

8. When completing a health risk appraisal the nurse should assess all of the following except

   A. personal health history.
   B. family health history.
   C. use of medications and drugs.
   *D. type of health insurance.

   Reference: p. 59

   Descriptors: 1. 04   2. 05   3. Application
                4. 2 = Assessment   5. Moderate

9. A client calling in to work in order to follow nursing orders to maintain bed rest is in what stage of illness behavior?

   A. Experiencing symptoms
   *B. Assuming sick role
   C. Assuming dependent role
   D. Achieving recovery and rehabilitation

   Reference: p. 60

   Descriptors: 1. 04   2. 05   3. Application
                4. 3 = Analysis/Diag.   5. Easy

10. Chronic illness differs from acute illness in that chronic illness

    A. leaves no permanent damage.
    B. requires little to no adaptation for cure.
    C. is cured in a short period of time.
    *D. causes irreversible damage or change.

    Reference: p. 61

    Descriptors: 1. 04   2. 04   3. Application
                 4. 1 = No Process   5. Easy

11. Appropriate nursing interventions for clients experiencing chronic illness include all of the following except

    *A. providing treatment for eventual cure.
    B. assisting the client in activities of daily living as needed.
    C. encouraging venting of emotions such as anger and grief.
    D. modifying the environment to enhance self-care.

    Reference: p. 61

    Descriptors: 1. 04   2. 05   3. Application
                 4. 5 = Implementation   5. Difficult

12. Assisting clients with hypertension to follow a low-sodium diet is an example of which of the following types of preventive care?

    A. Primary
    B. Secondary
    *C. Tertiary
    D. Restorative

    Reference: p. 61

    Descriptors   1. 04   2. 06   3. Application
                     4. 5 = Implementation 5. Moderate

CHAPTER 5
Theoretical Base for Nursing Practice

1. Concepts are to theory as bricks are to _____.

   *A. house
   B. mason
   C. wood
   D. mortar

   Reference: p. 66

   Descriptors   1. 05   2. 01   3. Application
                    4. 1 = No Process   5. Moderate

2. The nurse who views the family as an open system that influences and is influenced by the community is utilizing which theoretical framework as a basis for practice?

   *A. General systems
   B. Stress/adaptation
   C. Developmental
   D. Health continuum

   Reference: p. 67

   Descriptors   1. 05   2. 01   3. Application
                    4. 1 = No Process   5. Moderate

3. Characteristics of nursing theories include

   A. narrow focus and specificity.
   B. assumed definitions of concepts.
   C. specially formulated technical language.
   *D. research generation.

   Reference: p. 67

   Descriptors   1. 05   2. 02   3. Factual
                    4. 1 = No Process   5. Easy

4. Which of the following is not considered a common component of nursing theory?

   A. Man
   *B. Science
   C. Environment
   D. Health

   Reference: pp. 67–68

   Descriptors   1. 05   2. 04   3. Application
                    4. 1 = No Process   5. Moderate

5. Nightingale's influence in nursing is still felt in the following areas except

   A. research generation.
   B. theory development.
 *C. psychomotor skill development.
   D. nursing philosophy.

Reference: p. 68

Descriptors 1. 05   2. 04   3. Application
           4. 1 = No Process   5. Moderate

6. Which of the following is an example of how nursing theory advances nursing as a profession?

   A. Providing guidance in disease treatment and cure
   B. Increasing knowledge base of pharmacotherapeutics
   C. Increasing nursing's connection to other health care disciplines
 *D. Articulating concepts central to nursing to nurses

Reference: p. 69

Descriptors: 1. 05   2. 05   3. Application
           4. 1 = No Process   5. Moderate

7. A nurse who views clients as being embedded in a sociocultural environment while expressing self within those parameters utilizes which of the following theories?

   A. Johnson
 *B. Leininger
   C. Neuman
   D. Watson

Reference: pp. 70–71

Descriptors 1. 05   2. 05   3. Application
           4. 1 = No Process   5. Moderate

8. The nursing theory that states a person is a holistic being in constant interaction with the environment, behaving in predictable patterns within unique experiences is

   A. King.
   B. Neuman.
 *C. Rogers.
   D. Roy.

Reference: pp. 72–74

Descriptors 1. 05   2. 05   3. Application
           4. 1 = No Process   5. Moderate

9. A nurse utilizing Watson's theory when caring for terminally ill clients would

   A. focus on self-care abilities and deficits.
   B. assist clients in adapting to biopsychosocial changes.
 *C. provide comfort measures to assist the client to achieve optimal hope.
   D. promote a sense of balance between internal and external environments.

Reference: p. 75

Descriptors 1. 05   2. 05   3. Application
           4. 5 = Implementation 5. Moderate

CHAPTER 6
Values and Ethics in Nursing

1. A child repeating sayings heard from the parents is an example of what common mode of value transmission?

 *A. Modeling
   B. Moralizing
   C. Laissez-faire
   D. Responsible choice

Reference: p. 79

Descriptors: 1. 06   2. 02   3. Application
           4. 1 = No Process   5. Easy

2. When utilizing the responsible choice mode of value transmission with teenagers, an appropriate nursing intervention would be to instruct the parents to

   A. ground the teenager when returning late from activity.
   B. wear safety belts in car.
 *C. provide various viewpoints with discussion.
   D. enroll the teenager in a religious-sponsored high school.

Reference: p. 79

Descriptors: 1. 06   2. 02   3. Application
           4. 5 = Implementation 5. Moderate

3. After careful deliberation, a client decides to maintain her pregnancy. This is an example of which step in the value process?

 *A. Freely choosing from alternatives
   B. Prizing with pride and happiness
   C. Acting with consistency and regularity
   D. Respecting one's religious beliefs

Reference: p. 81

Descriptors: 1. 06   2. 04   3. Application
           4. 1 = No Process   5. Moderate

4. A diabetic is consistently choosing menu items within the prescribed diet plan. This client is using which step in the value process?

    A. Freely choosing from alternatives
    B. Understanding the probable consequences of non-compliance
    C. Taking pride in following diet regimen
    *D. Acting consistently on value of diet regimen

    Reference: p. 81

    Descriptors: 1. 06   2. 04   3. Application
                 4. 6 = Evaluation   5. Moderate

5. The nurse decides not to administer the medication due to possible untoward effects for the client. The nurse is acting upon which ethical conduct theory?

    *A. Nonmaleficence
    B. Deontologic
    C. Ethical
    D. Moral

    Reference: p. 83

    Descriptors: 1. 06   2. 01   3. Application
                 4. 1 = No Process   5. Moderate

6. When discussing the risks and benefits of a particular procedure with a client, the nurse is guided by which of the following approaches to ethical conduct?

    A. Autonomy
    B. Nonmaleficence
    *C. Utilitarian
    D. Justice

    Reference: p. 83

    Descriptors: 1. 06   2. 05   3. Application
                 4. 1 = No Process   5. Moderate

7. The nurse concerned with providing adequate prenatal care to disadvantaged women is acting under which of the four characteristics of ethical conduct based on general principles?

    A. Autonomy
    B. Nonmaleficence
    C. Beneficence
    *D. Justice

    Reference: p. 83

    Descriptors: 1. 06   2. 05   3. Application
                 4. 1 = No Process   5. Moderate

8. An appropriate nursing intervention utilizing a care-based approach for ethical conduct is

    A. directing care directed solely to the client's admitting diagnosis.
    B. providing care with only assigned clients in mind.
    C. distancing self from clients to provide objective care.
    *D. providing safe, holistic individualized care to each client.

    Reference: pp. 83–84

    Descriptors: 1. 06   2. 05   3. Application
                 4. 5 = Implementation 5. Moderate

9. Which of the following demonstrates the role of the nurse advocate? The nurse

    A. follows hospital rules over extenuating client needs.
    *B. allows a client's underage child to visit.
    C. defers client's rights over medical needs.
    D. refuses to relay client's wishes to other health care providers.

    Reference: p. 84

    Descriptors: 1. 06   2. 06   3. Application
                 4. 5 = Implementation 5. Moderate

10. The nurse allowed the client to leave his dentures in place until he went into the operating room. This is an example of

    *A. advocacy.
    B. principle-based care.
    C. justice.
    D. moral reasoning.

    Reference: p. 84

    Descriptors: 1. 06   2. 06   3. Application
                 4. 1 = No Process   5. Moderate

11. Which of the following nursing actions does not reflect ethical behavior as outlined in the nursing code of ethics?

    A. Keeping the client's chart in a safe place
    B. Refusing to discuss client's condition in public areas
    C. Providing safe, effective care to all clients equally
    *D. Upholding institutional regulations over the clients' needs and good

    Reference: p. 84

    Descriptors: 1. 06   2. 07   3. Application
                 4. 1 = No Process   5. Moderate

12. Which of the following statements reflects an ethical action by the nurse as described in the nursing code of ethics?

    A. "Did you hear about the client's daughter in 1315B?"
    B. "It's not my job to ask Dr. Smith to allow you to visit your new baby in the NICU."
  *C. "I understand your need to see your new grandchild. Let me see what I can do."
    D. "You know all of 'those people' are like that."

Reference: p. 84

Descriptors: 1. 06   2. 07   3. Application
               4. 1 = No Process   5. Moderate

13. A new mother tells the nurse that her husband is not the client's father and requests that the nurse only verbally communicate this information to the physician caring for the client. The infant is ill with a rare, inherited genetic disease. This dilemma is an example of

    A. paternalism.
    B. conflict of interest.
    C. deception.
  *D. confidentiality.

Reference: pp. 86–88

Descriptors: 1. 06   2. 08   3. Application
               4. 1 = No Process   5. Moderate

14. An illiterate client is awaiting surgery. The nurse obtains the client's signature on the surgical permit without verbal discussion of the procedure. This is an example of an ethical dilemma involving

  *A. informed consent.
    B. paternalism.
    C. confidentiality.
    D. deception.

Reference: pp. 86–88

Descriptors: 1. 06   2. 08   3. Application
               4. 1 = No Process   5. Moderate

15. Refusal to care for a client who failed at a suicide attempt is an example of which ethical dilemma?

    A. Paternalism
  *B. Conflict of interests or rights
    C. Allocation of scarce resources
    D. Confidentiality

Reference: pp. 86–88

Descriptors: 1. 06   2. 08   3. Application
               4. 1 = No Process   5. Moderate

16. Which of the following is an example of paternalistic behavior?

    A. Telling a client that a painful procedure doesn't hurt
    B. Deciding to close a telemetry unit when no monitored beds are left
  *C. Intercepting a visitor's gift of candy for a diabetic client
    D. Discussing the client's condition with another client

Reference: pp. 86–88

Descriptors: 1. 06   2. 08   3. Application
               4. 1 = No Process   5. Moderate

17. A nurse in the emergency room is caring for a client who is unable to speak or read English. The client requires emergency surgery. The client came to the hospital alone. The nurse should first

    A. schedule the surgery.
  *B. call an interpreter.
    C. determine the client's blood type.
    D. start an intravenous infusion.

Reference: p. 86

Descriptors: 1. 06   2. 09   3. Application
               4. 5 = Implementation 5. Difficult

18. A client who requires surgery but cannot speak English represents which of the following types of ethical dilemmas?

  *A. Inappropriate or inadequate informed consent was obtained.
    B. Surgeon has a religious conflict of interest with the client.
    C. A breach of client confidentiality has occurred.
    D. Scarcity of appropriate nursing resources is jeopardizing client care.

Reference: p. 86

Descriptors: 1. 06   2. 09   3. Application
               4. 3 = Analysis/Diag.   5. Difficult

19. An appropriate intervention for an underage client who is alone that requires emergency surgery would be

    A. procuring the services of a surgeon.
    B. withholding life-sustaining care until parents arrive.
    C. have the client sign an informed consent.
  *D. maintain patient airway and IV lines.

Reference: p. 86

Descriptors: 1. 06   2. 09   3. Application
               4. 5 = Implementation 5. Difficult

20. The nurse is caring for a client who requires surgery but cannot speak English. This ethical dilemma would be successfully resolved when

A. client and surgeon agree on appropriateness of surgical intervention.
*B. client understands risks and benefits of emergency procedure.
C. additional nursing assistance is given and safe care rendered to all clients.
D. client's condition is kept confidential throughout hospital stay.

Reference: p. 86

Descriptors: 1. 06   2. 09   3. Interpretive
              4. 6 = Evaluation   5. Difficult

21. After being notified by the nurse, a physician writes a resuscitation order for a client who has a current living will with detailed "do not resuscitate" orders. The physician's written orders are in direct opposition to the client's living will. This is an example of

A. deception over proposed medical regimen.
*B. disagreement over proposed medical regimen.
C. physician incompetence or malpractice.
D. conflict regarding the scope of nursing practice.

Reference: p. 91

Descriptors: 1. 06   2. 08   3. Application
              4. 1 = No Process   5. Moderate

22. A common ethical dilemma between nurse practitioners and physicians is

A. client deception.
B. scarcity of health care resources.
C. claims of loyalty.
*D. conflicts regarding the scope of nursing practice.

Reference: pp. 91–92

Descriptors: 1. 06   2. 08   3. Application
              4. 1 = No Process   5. Moderate

23. A nurse manager notes a discrepancy in the narcotic count. The manager finds a staff nurse in the locker room with the missing narcotic and a syringe. The staff nurse confides about the addiction, and asks for silence. This is an example of which ethical dilemma?

A. Nurse malpractice
B. Personal moral convictions versus practice demand
*C. Claims of loyalty between colleagues
D. Professional fraud

Reference: p. 92

Descriptors: 1. 06   2. 08   3. Application
              4. 1 = No Process   5. Moderate

24. The primary function of a health care institution ethics committee is to

*A. provide staff development about ethical decision-making.
B. enforce regulations set forth by the institution.
C. revoke professional licensure as appropriate.
D. provide legal services to clients and professionals.

Reference: p. 92

Descriptors: 1. 06   2. 10   3. Application
              4. 1 = No Process   5. Moderate

CHAPTER 7
Legal Implications in Nursing

1. Nurse practice acts are an example of which type of law?

A. Constitutional
*B. Statutory
C. Administrative
D. Common

Reference: p. 96

Descriptors: 1. 07   2. 02   3. Application
              4. 1 = No Process   5. Easy

2. Laws governing malpractice are which type of law?

A. Public
*B. Civil
C. Constitutional
D. Statutory

Reference: p. 96

Descriptors: 1. 07   2. 01   3. Application
              4. 1 = No Process   5. Easy

3. An example of a voluntary standard for nursing is

A. licensure.
B. nurse practice acts.
C. state boards of nursing.
*D. accreditation of educational programs.

Reference: p. 97

Descriptors: 1. 07   2. 03   3. Application
              4. 1 = No Process   5. Moderate

4. Which of the following statements is not true concerning professional and legal regulatory processes?

*A. State nurse practice acts are a product of professional regulation.
B. Professional regulation is voluntary.
C. Legal regulation covers licensure.
D. Public protection is the aim of legal regulation.

Reference: pp. 97–98

Descriptors: 1. 07   2. 03   3. Application
              4. 1 = No Process   5. Moderate

5. Which of the following is necessary for a nurse to practice nursing?

   A. Accreditation
   B. Certification
   C. Credentialing
 *D. Licensure

Reference: p. 98

Descriptors: 1. 07   2. 04   3. Application
          4. 1 = No Process 5. Easy

6. Nurse licensure and registration is earned upon

   A. graduation from an NLN-accredited school.
 *B. passing the licensing exam.
   C. completion of certification process.
   D. registering to practice in a specific state.

Reference: p. 98

Descriptors: 1. 07   2. 04   3. Application
          4. 1 = No Process 5. Moderate

7. Appropriate reasons for license revocation include

 *A. theft.
   B. bankruptcy.
   C. pregnancy.
   D. hearing impairment.

Reference: p. 98

Descriptors: 1. 07   2. 05   3. Application
          4. 1 = No Process 5. Moderate

8. The most common reason for registration or licensure revocation is

 *A. drug or alcohol abuse.
   B. fraud.
   C. deception.
   D. physical impairment.

Reference: p. 98

Descriptors: 1. 07   2. 04   3. Factual
          4. 1 = No Process 5. Easy

9. Accidental overdose may be considered what type of crime?

   A. Assault
   B. Battery
   C. Defamation of character
 *D. Negligence

Reference: p. 99

Descriptors: 1. 07   2. 06   3. Application
          4. 1 = No Process 5. Moderate

10. Inability to procure an informed consent prior to care rendered may result in what type of crime?

   A. Defamation of character
   B. Negligence
 *C. Battery
   D. Assault

Reference: p. 99

Descriptors: 1. 07   2. 06   3. Application
          4. 1 = No Process 5. Moderate

11. An appropiate nursing intervention to prevent a possible battery charge is to

 *A. obtain informed consent prior to performing procedures.
   B. obtain informed consent once procedures are completed.
   C. maintain a courteous, professional attitude at the workplace.
   D. encourage the client to sign all consent forms as soon as possible.

Reference: p. 99

Descriptors: 1. 07   2. 06   3. Application
          4. 5 = Implementation 5. Moderate

12. Which of the following is a possible risk factor in obtaining an informed consent?

   A. A client states understanding of medical condition.
 *B. A client is medicated for pain one hour prior to signing consent.
   C. A nurse understands the client's condition and rationale for procedure.
   D. The environment is pressure-free for client decision-making.

Reference: pp. 99–100

Descriptors: 1. 07   2. 06   3. Application
          4. 2 = Assessment 5. Moderate

13. An appropriate nursing intervention to prevent possible invasion of client privacy is to

   A. assess the client's verbal and written command of the English language.
 *B. request only necessary information for safe and effective care.
   C. promote a stress-free environment for decision-making.
   D. chart only factual information that is written or discussed.

Reference: p. 100

Descriptors: 1. 07   2. 06   3. Application
          4. 5 = Implementation 5. Moderate

14. Which of the following statements is false?

   A. A nurse can be sued for failure to obtain a written informed consent prior to completing a procedure.
   B. Careless discussion of a client's condition can be considered an invasion of privacy.
 *C. Once signed, an informed consent cannot be rescinded.
   D. Placing a client in restraints may be considered false imprisonment.

Reference: pp. 99–101

Descriptors: 1. 07   2. 06, 07 3. Interpretive
          4. 1 = No Process 5. Moderate

15. Failing to raise the siderails on the crib of a toddler can be considered what type of tort crime?

A. Battery
B. Fraud
C. False imprisonment
*D. Negligence

Reference: pp. 99–101

Descriptors: 1. 07   2. 06, 07   3. Application
4. 1 = No Process   5. Moderate

16. A client fell and sustained injuries while the bed was in the highest position. Proving a causal relationship is an example of which element of liability?

A. Duty
B. Breach of duty
*C. Causation
D. Damages

Reference: p. 101

Descriptors: 1. 07   2. 06   3. Application
4. 1 = No Process   5. Moderate

17. Which of the following is not a recommended action if a nurse is named a defendant in a lawsuit?

A. Do not discuss the case outside of legal counsel.
B. Maintain an open and honest relationship with legal counsel.
C. Do not volunteer any information.
*D. Alter records as necessary to correct deficiencies.

Reference: p. 102

Descriptors: 1. 07   2. 08   3. Application
4. 1 = No Process   5. Easy

18. Staff nurses can take part in legal proceedings in all of the following roles except

A. defendant.
B. fact witness.
C. expert witness.
*D. legal counsel.

Reference: p. 102

Descriptors: 1. 07   2. 09   3. Application
4. 1 = No Process   5. Easy

19. A nurse is subpoened to recall events of a particular client's hospitalization. The nurse is serving as a/an

A. defendant.
*B. fact witness.
C. expert witness.
D. plaintiff.

Reference: p. 102

Descriptors: 1. 07   2. 09   3. Application
4. 1 = No Process   5. Easy

20. Which of the following nurses can best serve as an expert witness in a malpractice suit involving surgery?

A. Graduate nurse working in the operating room 6 months
*B. Certified nurse working in the operating room 5 years
C. Charge nurse working in the emergency room 10 years
D. Staff nurse working in the operating room 5 years

Reference: p. 102

Descriptors: 1. 07   2. 09   3. Interpretive
4. 1 = No Process   5. Moderate

21. An example of potential liability in nursing assessment is a failure to

*A. detect change in the client's condition.
B. formulate a correct nursing diagnosis.
C. be sensitive to client's perceived needs.
D. implement prioritized interventions.

Reference: p. 103

Descriptors: 1. 07   2. 07   3. Application
4. 2 = Assessment   5. Moderate

22. The nurse fails to review the current nursing intervention for a client, resulting in a failure to resolve a priority problem. This is an example of a potential liability in which area of the nursing process?

A. Assessment
B. Diagnosis
C. Planning
*D. Evaluation

Reference: p. 103

Descriptors: 1. 07   2. 07   3. Application
4. 1 = No Process   5. Moderate

23. Failure to plan for potential client problems is an example of a potential liability in which area of the nursing process?

A. Assessment
B. Diagnosis
*C. Outcome identification
D. Planning

Reference: p. 103

Descriptors: 1. 07   2. 07   3. Application
4. 1 = No Process   5. Moderate

24. Failure to ensure that the client has full understanding of postoperative care needs that can result in client injury is an example of a potential liability in which area of the nursing process?

A. Assessment
B. Diagnosis
C. Planning
*D. Evaluation

Reference: pp. 103–104

Descriptors: 1. 07   2. 07   3. Application
4. 1 = No Process   5. Moderate

25. Which of the following reflects a failure in collecting an accurate client health database?

  A. Labeling an obese client as noncompliant with medical regimen
  B. Failure to teach the parents of a 2-year-old head trauma victim the signs of increasing intercranial pressure
 *C. Failure to report low blood sugar results on a diabetic client to resident on call
  D. Failure to relay client's "do not resuscitate" wishes as stated in the living will to the physician

Reference: pp. 103–104

Descriptors: 1. 07   2. 07   3. Application
               4. 1 = No Process   5. Moderate

26. Examples of maintaining a competent nursing practice include all of the following except

  A. following institutional policies and procedures.
  B. attending relevant educational opportunities.
  C. maintaining licensure.
 *D. accepting client cases outside of specialty area.

References: p. 104

Descriptors: 1. 07   2. 10   3. Application
               4. 1 = No Process   5. Moderate

27. Which of the following statements denotes a failure to adequately provide client education?

  A. Utilizing a variety of tools to promote a full understanding of the teaching need
  B. Maintaining a current and acceptable practice
  C. Teaching family members as deemed appropriate
 *D. Not documenting teaching provided

Reference: pp. 104–105

Descriptors: 1. 07   2. 07   3. Application
               4. 4 = Planning   5. Moderate

28. Which of the following statements is false regarding litigation for negligence?

 *A. A trial occurs whether or not the arbitration panel's decision is accepted by all parties.
  B. A malpractice arbitration panel reviews the case for relevancy.
  C. Defendants can accept or reject offers for settlements.
  D. All elements for liability need to be present for malpractice suits to go to trial.

Reference: pp. 102–105

Descriptors: 1. 07   2. 08   3. Application
               4. 1 = No Process   5. Moderate

29. The purpose of incident reports includes all of the following except

 *A. a substitute for documentation on the client's chart.
  B. documentation of potential harm to anyone within the institution.
  C. identification of actual and potential risks.
  D. treatment and management of client problems.

Reference: p. 108

Descriptors: 1. 07   2. 11   3. Application
               4. 1 = No Process   5. Easy

30. A nurse providing CPR in an apparent cardiac arrest in an accident victim is protected under which general set of laws?

  A. Nurse practice
 *B. Good Samaritan
  C. Occupational safety and health
  D. Health care quality improvement

Reference: pp. 108–110

Descriptors: 1. 07   2. 12   3. Application
               4. 1 = No Process   5. Easy

UNIT II
PROMOTING WELLNESS ACROSS THE LIFE SPAN

CHAPTER 8
Developmental Concepts

1. Which of the following is not a general principle of growth and development?

   A. Children learn to walk before learning to run.
   *B. Genetics determines level of developmental maturity.
   C. Head control occurs before hand clapping.
   D. An ill child may experience delayed puberty.

   Reference: pp. 115–117

   Descriptors: 1. 08   2. 01, 02   3. Application
                4. 1 = No Process   5. Easy

2. Few children are able to be equally adept at academics and athletics due to

   A. predictable patterns of growth and development.
   B. cephalocaudal development.
   C. inability to modify growth and development.
   *D. temporary concentration of energies on one skill.

   Reference: pp. 115–117

   Descriptors: 1. 08   2. 02   3. Application
                4. 1 = No Process   5. Easy

3. A teenager who is actively maintaining her own virginity until marriage is considered to be in which of Freud's stages of psychosocial development?

   A. Unconscious mind, latent stage
   B. Id, latent stage
   C. Ego, genital stage
   *D. Superego, genital stage

   Reference: p. 117

   Descriptors: 1. 08   2. 03   3. Interpretive
                4. 3 = Analysis/Diag.   5. Moderate

4. An adult is unable to form relationships due to underlying inability to trust. This may be due to an unsuccessful resolution of which stage of Erickson's developmental theory?

   *A. Trust versus mistrust
   B. Identity versus role confusion
   C. Intimacy versus isolation
   D. Generativity versus stagnation

   Reference: pp. 117–118

   Descriptors: 1. 08   2. 03   3. Interpretive
                4. 3 = Analysis/Diag.   5. Moderate

5. Nursing's code of ethics requires nurses to provide holistic care for all clients. This is an example of which of the following stages of Kohlberg and Gilligan's moral development?

   A. Social contract, utilitarian
   *B. Universal ethical principle
   C. Law and order
   D. Instrumental relativist

   Reference: pp. 119–121

   Descriptors: 1. 08   2. 03   3. Interpretive
                4. 3 = Analysis/Diag.   5. Easy

6. The ability to apply the nursing process and critically think through client care situations requires which stage of Piaget's theory on cognitive development?

   A. Sensorimotor
   B. Preoperational
   C. Concrete operational
   *D. Formal operational

   Reference: p. 119

   Descriptors: 1. 08   2. 03   3. Interpretive
                4. 3 = Analysis/Diag.   5. Easy

7. Gilligan's feminist theory of moral development is in agreement with nursing philosophy because it provides for

   A. creation of equal rights for all.
   B. promotion of following societal norms and mores.
   *C. universal promotion of holistic welfare.
   D. internal sense of justice for society.

   Reference: pp. 121–122

   Descriptors: 1. 08   2. 03   3. Application
                4. 1 = No Process   5. Moderate

8. When discussing values and beliefs, a client states, "I've decided that the faith I grew up with isn't the one that I believe in. I have found and now attend a new church and am very happy." The client is working through which phase of Fowler's faith development?

   A. Stage 2: mythical-ethical
   B. Stage 3: synthetic-conventional
   *C. Stage 4: individual-reflective
   D. Stage 5: conjunctive

   Reference: pp. 122–123

   Descriptors: 1. 08   2. 03   3. Interpretive
                4. 3 = Analysis/Diag.   5. Moderate

9. Which of the following statements should guide developing a program to teach adolescents how to inject insulin? Adolescents

   *A. may help gain a sense of role identity by working with other diabetic teens.
   B. will not be concerned about peer opinion.
   C. are concerned with achieving independence from peers and parents.
   D. are not able to understand the consequences of noncompliance.

   Reference: pp. 125–127

   Descriptors: 1. 08   2. 04   3. Interpretive
                4. 1 = No Process   5. Moderate

10. A 2-year-old cries every day when left at the day care center. The nurse should tell the parent that the child

    A. can be reasoned with in a logical manner.
    B. is experiencing a severe emotional trauma and needs help.
    C. is deliberately trying to induce guilt and the behavior should be ignored.
    *D. is experiencing a normal learning phase and will soon grow out of it.

    Reference: pp. 125–127

    Descriptors: 1. 08   2. 04   3. Application
                 4. 5 = Implementation 5. Moderate

11. In assisting a middle-aged couple care for an elderly parent, the nurse explains that older adults are in the process of achieving which of the following developmental tasks?

    *A. Accepting the changes that accompany the aging process
    B. Earning an income
    C. Assisting children to become well-adjusted adults
    D. Preparing for death

    Reference: pp. 125–127

    Descriptors: 1. 08   2. 04   3. Application
                 4. 5 = Implementation 5. Easy

12. A nurse is teaching an 8-year-old to give insulin. The nurse should inform the parents that

    A. severe stress will cause a premature "jump" into the next developmental level.
    B. mild stress may result in the loss of bowel and bladder control.
    *C. hesitancy may occur when learning new skills.
    D. concern over body image and sexual relationships may intensify.

    Reference: pp. 125–127

    Descriptors: 1. 08   2. 05   3. Application
                 4. 5 = Implementation 5. Moderate

13. To effectively care for the paraplegic teen, which of the following family data would be most helpful?

    A. Teen's personal and medical history; presence of allergies
    *B. Parents' occupations; home structure, ages of siblings
    C. Teen's academic record, likes and dislikes; parental attitude
    D. Teen's relationships with peers; parents' socioeconomic status

    Reference: pp. 125–127

    Descriptors: 1. 08   2. 05, 06   3. Interpretive
                 4. 2 = Assessment   5. Moderate

CHAPTER 9
Conception Through Adolescence

1. During which prenatal time period is the unborn at greatest risk for anomalies due to teratogenic exposure?

   A. Conception
   *B. Pre-embryonic
   C. Embryonic
   D. Fetal

   Reference: pp. 129–130

   Descriptors: 1. 09   2. 02   3. Factual
                4. 1 = No Process   5. Easy

2. Maturation of organs and body systems in preparation for extrauterine life occurs during which prenatal time period?

   A. Conception
   B. Pre-embryonic
   C. Embryonic
   *D. Fetal

   Reference: pp. 129–130

   Descriptors: 1. 09   2. 02   3. Factual
                4. 1 = No Process   5. Easy

3. The nurse can teach the new parent that their neonate is able to do all of the following except

   A. suckle from bottle or breast.
   B. differentiate between the mother and others by smell.
   *C. shiver and sweat to maintain thermoregulation.
   D. turn eyes in direction of noise.

   Reference: pp. 130–134

   Descriptors: 1. 09   2. 02, 03   3. Application
                4. 5 = Implementation 5. Moderate

4. Which of the following is most immediately life-threatening to a neonate?

  *A. APGAR score of three
  B. Physiologic jaundice
  C. Molding
  D. Cocaine addiction

  Reference: pp. 130–134

  Descriptors: 1. 09   2. 03   3. Interpretive
               4. 3 = Analysis/Diag.   5. Moderate

5. Long-term growth and development effects are most likely to occur in the neonate affected with

  A. caput succedaneum.
  B. subconjunctival henorrhage.
  C. physiologic jaundice.
  *D. fetal alcohol syndrome

  Reference: pp. 130–134

  Descriptors: 1. 09   2. 03   3. Interpretive
               4. 3 = Analysis/Diag.   5. Moderate

6. The largest physiologic growth period occurs during which of the following stages?

  *A. Infancy
  B. Preschooler
  C. School age
  D. Adolescence

  Reference: pp. 130–134

  Descriptors: 1. 09   2. 02   3. Factual
               4. 2 = Assessment   5. Easy

7. Nursing actions to promote health and wellness in infants include

  A. keeping a large assortment of small toys in the crib at all times.
  B. maintaining a quiet, dark environment for adequate sleep.
  *C. checking the infant when crying occurs.
  D. allowing the infant to verbalize by prolonged crying.

  Reference: pp. 130–134

  Descriptors: 1. 09   2. 04   3. Application
               4. 5 = Implementation 5. Moderate

8. Appropriate child care items for toddlers typically include

  *A. pull toys and training pants.
  B. drinking glasses and crayons.
  C. car seats and bicycles.
  D. hard candies and electric outlet covers.

  Reference: pp. 134–138

  Descriptors: 1. 09   2. 04   3. Application
               4. 4 = Planning   5. Moderate

9. Appropriate teaching principles to discuss with parents of toddlers include

  A. providing rationale to the toddler when disciplining for bad behavior.
  B. discipline is necessary when a toddler cries when separated from the parents.
  *C. safe placement of household cleaners is vital for safety.
  D. hard candies and sweets will calm a crying toddler.

  Reference: pp. 134–138

  Descriptors: 1. 09   2. 03, 04   3. Application
               4. 4 = Planning   5. Moderate

10. Caring for preschoolers includes all of the following nursing actions except

  A. being honest about painful procedures.
  *B. asking the child for permission before giving an injection.
  C. explaining how the incision will look after surgery.
  D. allowing the parents to stay with the child preoperatively.

  Reference: pp. 138–140

  Descriptors: 1. 09   2. 04   3. Application
               4. 5 = Implementation 5. Moderate

11. In teaching wellness and health promotion to parents of school-aged children, discussion should include

  *A. wearing helmets while roller-blading.
  B. visiting the dentist every other year.
  C. encouraging diets high in fats.
  D. using antibiotics to prevent sexually transmitted diseases.

  Reference: pp. 140–142

  Descriptors: 1. 09   2. 04   3. Application
               4. 5 = Implementation 5. Moderate

12. The nurse is discussing play toys with the parents of school-aged children. Appropriate play toys for school-aged children include

  A. blocks.
  B. mobiles.
  *C. bicycles.
  D. pull toys.

  Reference: pp. 140–142

  Descriptors: 1. 09   2. 02, 04   3. Interpretive
               4. 5 = Implementation 5. Easy

13. Adolescence is a challenging period for both teens and caregivers. The main reason for this is the

   A. emergence of self-acceptance.
   B. decision-making for career roles.
   C. development of mature relationships with peers.
   *D. striving for independence from caregivers.

   Reference: pp. 142–148

   Descriptors: 1. 09   2. 02, 04   3. Application
                4. 1 = No Process   5. Easy

14. Beliefs that increase the likelihood of nutritional difficulties in adolescents include all of the following needs except for

   A. acceptance by peers.
   B. achievement of success in school.
   C. control of their environment.
   *D. decreased need for calories.

   Reference: pp. 142–148

   Descriptors: 1. 09   2. 02, 04   3. Application
                4. 3 = Analysis/Diag.   5. Moderate

15. Nursing actions appropriate for the resolution of the nursing diagnosis "Potential for infection, related to indiscriminate sexual activity" for adolescents include

   A. providing medical treatments.
   *B. teaching transmission mode of infections.
   C. advising clients to curtail their sexual activities.
   D. contacting caregivers about their sexual activity.

   Reference: pp. 142–148

   Descriptors: 1. 09   2. 02, 04   3. Interpretive
                4. 5 = Implementation 5. Moderate

CHAPTER 10
Early, Middle, and Older Adulthood

1. A developmental task for a 45-year-old client is the

   A. development of a sense of independence.
   *B. acceptance of "wrinkles and gray hair."
   C. establishment of a personal philosophy.
   D. establishment of peer and intimate relationships.

   Reference: pp. 150–151

   Descriptors: 1. 10   2. 02   3. Application
                4. 2 = Assessment   5. Easy

2. A similarity between Levison's and Gould's adult developmental theories is that

   A. physiological changes are the basis of these theories.
   B. changes between stages occur in isolation.
   *C. biopsychosocial changes occur along the life's continuum.
   D. deterioration of life occurs after the age of 50.

   Reference: pp. 150–151

   Descriptors: 1. 10   2. 02   3. Interpretive
                4. 1 = No Process   5. Easy

3. An appropriate nursing action to assist those involved to successfully accomplish the tasks of pregnancy include all of the following except to

   A. help those involved accept or reject the pregnancy.
   B. provide holistic woman and infant care information.
   C. inform the family of the woman's special needs.
   *D. advise the client and family of the nurse's values and beliefs.

   Reference: pp. 152–154

   Descriptors: 1. 10   2. 03, 07   3. Interpretive
                4. 5 = Implementation 5. Moderate

4. Nursing actions to promote health for young adults include all of the following except

   A. providing assistance for coping with multiple roles.
   *B. giving advice on child-rearing.
   C. providing information on community resources.
   D. teaching the importance of preventative health.

   Reference: pp. 152–154

   Descriptors: 1. 10   2. 04, 07   3. Interpretive
                4. 5 = Implementation 5. Moderate

5. Nursing actions to assist adult clients in coping with the stressors associated with role transition include

   *A. discussing stressors with the family and health care providers.
   B. advising clients to seek professional assistance as needed.
   C. prescribing antidepressants for stress-related symptoms.
   D. providing psychotherapy for severely stressed clients.

   Reference: pp. 154–155

   Descriptors: 1. 10   2. 04, 07   3. Application
                4. 5 = Implementation 5. Moderate

6. Myths surrounding ageism commonly held by nurses include

   *A. senility.
   B. sexuality.
   C. coping.
   D. adapting.

   Reference: pp. 165–166

   Descriptors: 1. 10   2. 01, 08   3. Factual
                4. 1 = No Process   5. Easy

7. Truths about aging include which statement?

   A. Older men outnumber older women.
   B. Over one-half of the population of adults over 50 live in assisted housing.
   C. Few old-old require health care assistance.
   *D. Aging is an individual experience.

   Reference: pp. 165–166

   Descriptors: 1. 10   2. 01, 08   3. Factual
                4. 1 = No Process   5. Easy

8. Which of the following is true of the relationship between the physiologic and functional status in aging?

   A. There is no correlation between the two concepts.
   *B. Adaptation to abilities varies among individuals.
   C. Usually only one functional status is affected.
   D. No other factors affect this particular relationship.

   Reference: pp. 164–165

   Descriptors: 1. 10   2. 05   3. Application
                4. 1 = No Process   5. Easy

9. In caring for the older adult, the nurse should consider that

   *A. there is a decreased capacity to adapt to illness.
   B. senility is a common finding among the elderly.
   C. there is a need for increased dosages in medication.
   D. learning capabilities are diminished.

   Reference: pp. 166–170

   Descriptors: 1. 10   2. 02, 03, 04, 07, 09
                3. Application   4. 2 = Assessment
                5. Moderate

10. Reminiscence can assist the older adult in accomplishing which of Erikson's developmental tasks?

    A. Resolution of future failures and disappointments
    *B. Restructuring of achieved and yet-to-be-achieved accomplishments
    C. Maintaining a sense of self-indulgence
    D. Complete removal of past failures and problems

    Reference: pp. 166–170

    Descriptors: 1. 10   2. 01, 07   3. Application
                 4. 1 = No Process   5. Moderate

11. Resources that nurses can identify to assist the older clients in achieving Havighurst's developmental tasks include all of the following except

    A. volunteer work at the local hospital.
    B. Visiting Nurse Association and Hospice organizations.
    C. Welfare, Meals-on-Wheels, and Medicaid programs.
    *D. Women, Infants and Children program.

    Reference: pp. 161–162

    Descriptors: 1. 10   2. 03, 09   3. Interpretive
                 4. 4 = Planning   5. Moderate

12. Nursing actions to promote wellness or prevent illness in the elderly include

    A. administering antidepressants for unresolved grief.
    *B. teaching the importance of nutrition and exercise.
    C. advising eliminating strenuous activity to decrease the risk of injury.
    D. using restraints while sleeping.

    Reference: pp. 164–170

    Descriptors: 1. 10   2. 07, 09   3. Application
                 4. 5 = Implementation 5. Moderate

13. Nursing actions to assist the elderly in preventing falls include

    A. avoiding unnecessary ambulation.
    B. decreasing room lighting to reduce possible glare.
    *C. removing rugs and debris from floors.
    D. decreasing amounts of all prescribed medications.

    Reference: pp. 164–170

    Descriptors: 1. 10   2. 07, 09   3. Application
                 4. 5 = Implementation 5. Moderate

14. Which of the following most adversely affects the elderly's ability to meet their needs?

    A. High cost of assisted living facilities.
    B. Lack of senior citizen programs.
    *C. Inadequate accessible public transportation.
    D. Consumer protection programs.

    Reference: pp. 161–164

    Descriptors: 1. 10   2. 06   3. Application
                 4. 1 = No Process   5. Easy

UNIT III
COMMUNITY-BASED SETTINGS FOR CLIENT CARE

CHAPTER 11
Community-Based Health Care

1. A community health nurse is planning a presentation to a group of high school students on nursing as a profession. Which of the following should be included in the teaching plan?

   *A. Home-based care is one of the most rapidly growing areas of the health care system.
   B. The number of advanced practice nurses is declining.
   C. The scope of nursing practice has been narrowed due to the number of other health care workers.
   D. Clients admitted to the hospital are usually severely ill and remain hospitalized for lengthy periods.

   Reference: p. 176

   Descriptors: 1. 11   2. 02   3. Factual
                4. 4 = Planning   5. Easy

2. The nurse has explained the goals of the Healthy People 2000 report to a group of beginning nursing students. The nurse determines that one of the students needs *further* instructions when he says that one of the goals is to

   A. decrease smoking for at least 60% of pregnant women.
   *B. reduce traffic deaths by 100% usage of car seats for infants.
   C. reduce the rise in deaths from COPD to no more than 25 per 100,000.
   D. decrease the number of children age 6 and younger who are exposed to tobacco smoke.

   Reference: p. 176

   Descriptors: 1. 11   2. 02   3. Factual
                4. 6 = Evaluation   5. Moderate

3. An adult client without health insurance will most likely receive care in a hospital that is termed

   A. public, for profit.
   B. private, for profit.
   C. private, not for profit.
   *D. public, not for profit.

   Reference: p. 177

   Descriptors: 1. 11   2. 01   3. Factual
                4. 1 = No Process   5. Easy

4. One of the major sources of emergency care and health education for children in the United States is nurses employed in

   A. ambulatory care centers.
   B. ambulatory surgery centers.
   C. hospital emergency rooms.
   *D. elementary and high schools.

   Reference: p. 179

   Descriptors: 1. 11   2. 04   3. Factual
                4. 1 = No Process   5. Easy

5. The nurse has presented a class on healthy lifestyles to a group of adults aged 65 and older. The nurse determines that one of the participants needs *further* instructions when he says that long-term care facilities have increased due to the

   *A. increased number of older adults with long-term care insurance.
   B. number of older adults who are living longer.
   C. lack of caregivers within the client's family.
   D. decreased length of hospital stays.

   Reference: p. 180

   Descriptors: 1. 11   2. 03   3. Application
                4. 6 = Evaluation   5. Moderate

6. The nurse is caring for a hospitalized client with a terminal illness who is expected to die within 3 months and who will be discharged soon. The nurse should assess the client for a possible referral to a

   A. rehabilitation center.
   B. long-term care facility.
   *C. hospice center.
   D. public health center.

   Reference: p. 180

   Descriptors: 1. 11   2. 04   3. Application
                4. 2 = Assessment   5. Moderate

7. The nurse is employed in a health care facility in which the cost-effective care of the client is carefully monitored from initial contact to discharge. This type of system is termed

   A. case management.
   B. primary health care.
   C. collaborative care.
   *D. managed care.

   Reference: p. 182

   Descriptors: 1. 11   2. 05   3. Factual
                4. 1 = No Process   5. Easy

8. The nurse is caring for a pregnant client who has decided to put her baby up for adoption. The nurse should refer the client to a

 *A. social worker.
  B. family planner.
  C. physician's assistant.
  D. chaplain.

Reference: p. 184

Descriptors: 1. 11   2. 06   3. Application
             4. 5 = Implementation 5. Easy

9. The nurse is caring for an adult client in the clinic when the client asks the nurse, "What is the difference between Health Maintenance Organizations and Preferred Provider Organizations?" The nurse's *best* response is to instruct the client that

  A. HMO's allow several choices of health care providers.
 *B. HMO's support the concept of managed care.
  C. PPO's do not allow the client to seek care from other providers outside the group.
  D. PPO's provide services at a higher fee to the insurer.

Reference: p. 186

Descriptors: 1. 11   2. 07   3. Application
             4. 5 = Implementation 5. Moderate

10. One of the major trends which will affect health care delivery over the next few years is the

  A. decreased emphasis on technology.
  B. increased emphasis on continuity of care.
  C. decreased competition among hospitals.
 *D. increased number of individuals over the age of 70.

Reference: p. 186

Descriptors: 1. 11   2. 08   3. Factual
             4. 1 = No Process   5. Easy

CHAPTER 12
Continuity of Care

1. The nurse has discussed continuity of care with a group of beginning nursing students. The nurse determines that one of the students needs *further* instructions when she says that continuity of care includes

  A. collaborating with other members of the health care team.
  B. discharge planning for any client who enters the health care system.
  C. involving the client and family in decisions related to care.
 *D. documenting the client's physical assessment findings.

Reference: p. 192

Descriptors: 1. 12   2. 01   3. Application
             4. 6 = Evaluation   5. Moderate

2. A client is scheduled to have surgery on his feet in an ambulatory surgery facility. Before the surgery is performed, the nurse should determine if the client

 *A. has had appropriate screening tests.
  B. has assistance from a family member at home.
  C. needs a bath or shower with Betadine soap.
  D. should be admitted to the hospital following surgery.

Reference: p. 194

Descriptors: 1. 12   2. 04   3. Application
             4. 2 = Assessment   5. Moderate

3. The nurse has assisted with the transfer of an adult client to a different unit in the hospital setting. Following the transfer, the nurse should

 *A. provide the receiving nurse with a verbal report.
  B. be certain the client's personal belongings have been sent home.
  C. ask the client to review the advance directives.
  D. provide the receiving nurse with the client's prescriptions.

Reference: p. 197

Descriptors: 1. 12   2. 05   3. Application
             4. 5 = Implementation 5. Moderate

4. To obtain an adult client's weight soon after admission to the hospital, the nurse should *first*

  A. ask the client to remove her shoes.
  B. move the sliding scale to the left.
  C. assist the client to step on the scale platform.
 *D. balance the scale on zero.

Reference: p. 200

Descriptors: 1. 12   2. 04   3. Application
             4. 5 = Implementation 5. Easy

5. The nurse has weighed an adult male client who is 6 feet tall with a medium frame. The client's weight is 170 pounds. The nurse determines that the client's weight is

  A. less than the recommended amount for a client who is 6 feet tall.
  B. more than the recommended amount for an adult male.
 *C. within normal limits for a medium-frame adult male.
  D. appropriate for a client with a small frame.

Reference: p. 200

Descriptors: 1. 12   2. 04   3. Interpretive
             4. 3 = Analysis/Diag. 5. Moderate

6. An adult client who has been hospitalized decides to leave the hospital against medical advice (AMA) and refuses to sign the release form. The nurse should

A. try to convince the client to remain hospitalized.
B. notify the hospital security department.
C. contact the hospital's legal department.
*D. document the explanation to the client in the medical record.

Reference: p. 201

Descriptors: 1. 12   2. 05   3. Application
     4. 5 = Implementation 5. Moderate

7. To insure continuity of care of a newly hospitalized client, the nurse initiates discharge planning for the client

*A. as soon as possible after admission.
B. within 48 hours after admission.
C. the day before discharge.
D. on the day of discharge.

Reference: p. 202

Descriptors: 1. 12   2. 06   3. Application
     4. 5 = Implementation 5. Easy

8. An adult client hospitalized for abdominal surgery will be dismissed to home in the morning. The nurse has instructed the client how to perform necessary dressing changes at home. Before the client is released the nurse should

A. ask the client to verbalize the procedure.
B. provide the client with a short quiz about the procedure.
C. determine if the client has any questions about his treatment plan.
*D. ask the client to perform a demonstration of the dressing change.

Reference: p. 203

Descriptors: 1. 12   2. 06   3. Application
     4. 5 = Implementation 5. Moderate

9. The nurse is preparing to discharge an adult client who will be using a wheelchair at home. An important assessment for the nurse to make is

A. who the caregiver will be when the client is home.
B. how often the client needs to have home care.
*C. whether the client's dwelling can accommodate a wheelchair.
D. whether or not the client has adequate insurance coverage.

Reference: p. 203

Descriptors: 1. 12   2. 06   3. Application
     4. 2 = Assessment   5. Moderate

10. A frail 86-year-old client will be dismissed from the hospital to home following a total knee replacement. In order for the client's home care referral to be reimbursed, the nurse should

*A. have a written order by the physician.
B. ask the social worker to document the client's needs.
C. have the client give her permission for home care.
D. document the client's home care needs in the medical record.

Reference: p. 205

Descriptors: 1. 12   2. 06   3. Application
     4. 5 = Implementation 5. Moderate

CHAPTER 13
Home Health Care

1. A major purpose of home health care is to

A. care for acutely ill clients.
B. promote self-care within the family.
C. rehabilitate clients who have had injuries.
*D. minimize the effects of illness and disability.

Reference: p. 208

Descriptors: 1. 13   2. 01   3. Factual
     4. 1 = No Process   5. Easy

2. In 1893 a home care agency established by Lillian Wald and Mary Brewster provided home care nurses to care for poor clients living in tenements. This was the beginning of the

*A. Visiting Nurse Association.
B. Public Health Nurses Association.
C. Home Health Care Nurses Association.
D. American Nurses Association.

Reference: p. 208

Descriptors: 1. 13   2. 02   3. Factual
     4. 1 = No Process   5. Easy

3. A major difference between nurses who work in an acute care setting and those employed in a home care agency is the nurse's

A. communication skills.
*B. independence.
C. technical skills.
D. reimbursement for services.

Reference: pp. 210–211

Descriptors: 1. 13   2. 03   3. Factual
     4. 1 = No Process   5. Easy

4. During the *Pre-entry* phase of the home visit, the nurse assigned to the client should plan to

A. negotiate the times of the visits.
B. develop detailed nursing care plans.
C. establish rapport with the client.
*D. gather information about the client.

Reference: p. 213

Descriptors: 1. 13   2. 04   3. Application
4. 4 = Planning   5. Moderate

5. During the *Entry* phase of the home visit, the nurse should

*A. determine desired outcomes with the client.
B. determine past surgical experiences.
C. gather necessary supplies for the client.
D. obtain a doctor's order for the visits.

Reference: p. 213

Descriptors: 1. 13   2. 04   3. Application
4. 5 = Implementation 5. Moderate

6. The home health nurse is caring for a client who is on a soft diet and immobilized due to partial paralysis. The client has several family members to care for her. A primary nursing diagnosis for this client is

A. Impaired social interaction related to injuries.
B. Risk for trauma related to immobility.
*C. Risk for constipation related to lack of dietary bulk.
D. Impaired skin integrity related to partial paralysis.

Reference: p. 215

Descriptors: 1. 13   2. 03   3. Application
4. 3 = Analysis/Diag.   5. Moderate

7. The nurse plans to assess a home health care client who is from a cultural group that is different from the nurse. To assess cultural factors related to activities of daily living the nurse should assess the client's

*A. nutritional practices.
B. sources of spiritual support.
C. beliefs about illness and therapies.
D. family structure and roles.

Reference: p. 216

Descriptors: 1. 13   2. 05   3. Application
4. 2 = Assessment   5. Moderate

8. The nurse is preparing to discharge an adult client from the hospital to home where the client's wife will be the major care provider for the client. One of the primary differences for family members between acute care and home care is that for clients in acute care settings, the family member

A. may not be competent to provide care.
B. has limited knowledge of the client's needs.
C. usually has limited skills for providing care.
*D. may become overwhelmed by the provision of care.

Reference: p. 217

Descriptors: 1. 13   2. 05   3. Application
4. 3 = Analysis/Diag.   5. Moderate

9. The nurse has explained hospice care to a family member of a client dying from cancer. The nurse determines that the family member understands the nurse's instructions when she says that hospice care

A. is most often provided in a hospice center.
B. begins when the client has 1 year to live.
*C. ends with the family 1 year after the death.
D. is not reimbursed by Medicare insurance.

Reference: p. 217

Descriptors: 1. 13   2. 06   3. Application
4. 6 = Evaluation   5. Moderate

10. If current trends in the United States continue, home health care will

*A. require more specialized nurses.
B. provide greater emphasis on illness care.
C. depend on nurses who are more generalized.
D. care for clients with less acuity than in the past.

Reference: p. 217

Descriptors: 1. 13   2. 02   3. Factual
4. 1 = No Process   5. Easy

UNIT IV
THE NURSING PROCESS

CHAPTER 14
Introduction to Nursing Process

1. The state board examination for licensure reflects the view that nursing has evolved to a

   A. more disease-based perspective.
   *B. holistic approach utilizing the nursing process.
   C. medical model approach.
   D. technologically based profession.

   Reference: p. 223

   Descriptors: 1. 14   2. 02   3. Factual
                  4. 1 = No Process   5. Easy

2. The steps of the nursing process include all of the following except

   A. assessing clients, communities, and families.
   *B. deriving a medical diagnosis for curing disease.
   C. planning care via mutual goal setting.
   D. evaluating the planned care response.

   Reference: pp. 223–226

   Descriptors: 1. 14   2. 03   3. Application
                  4. 1 = No Process   5. Moderate

3. The assessment step of the nursing process includes all of the following except

   A. gathering pertinent lab data.
   B. interviewing the client about present and past health concerns.
   C. upgrading the database as necessary.
   *D. revising the nursing diagnosis when appropriate.

   Reference: p. 225

   Descriptors: 1. 14   2. 01, 03   3. Factual
                  4. 2 = Assessment   5. Moderate

4. Successful resolution of the nursing goal "Client will remain free from injury during hospital stay" comprises

   *A. no falls recorded during hospital stay.
   B. range of motion normal for all joints.
   C. restraints used at night.
   D. siderails up while the client is in bed.

   Reference: pp. 225–226

   Descriptors: 1. 14   2. 01, 03   3. Application
                  4. 6 = Evaluation   5. Moderate

5. Characteristics of the nursing process include all of the following except

   A. logical.
   B. cyclic.
   *C. stagnant.
   D. generalizable.

   Reference: pp. 228–230

   Descriptors: 1. 14   2. 04   3. Application
                  4. 1 = No Process   5. Easy

6. Benefits for clients and nurses when the nursing process is utilized include care that is provided in which of the following ways?

   A. Ritualistic
   B. Standardized
   *C. Individualized
   D. Robotic

   Reference: p. 230

   Descriptors: 1. 14   2. 05   3. Factual
                  4. 1 = No Process   5. Easy

CHAPTER 15
Essential Knowledge and Skills in Nursing

1. The ability to safely and effectively utilize intravenous equipment is an example of which of the four basic skills necessary for nursing practice?

   A. Cognitive
   *B. Technical
   C. Interpersonal
   D. Ethical/legal

   Reference: pp. 233–235

   Descriptors: 1. 15   2. 02   3. Application
                  4. 1 = No Process   5. Moderate

2. Maintaining a trusting and accountable relationship with clients and other health care professionals is an example of which of the four basic skills necessary for nursing practice?

   A. Cognitive
   B. Technical
   C. Interpersonal
   *D. Ethical/legal

   Reference: pp. 233–235

   Descriptors: 1. 15   2. 02   3. Application
                  4. 1 = No Process   5. Moderate

3. A student nurse is learning to don sterile gloves. Which of the following will be most helpful to the student in mastering the skill?

   A. Reflecting on potential ethical dilemmas
   B. Watching a videotape of the procedure
  *C. Practicing the technique in the learning lab
   D. Listing personal strengths and weaknesses

Reference: pp. 236–241

Descriptors: 1. 15   2. 04   3. Application
             4. 1 = No Process   5. Moderate

4. All of the following are appropriate interventions for enhancing communication skills except

   A. practicing various communication skills with peers.
   B. using an audio record of conversations with peers to review skills.
   C. reflecting on personal biases.
  *D. reviewing the procedure prior to implementation.

Reference: pp. 236–241

Descriptors: 1. 15   2. 05   3. Application
             4. 5 = Implementation 5. Moderate

5. A nurse leaves the unit without reporting to the designated relief colleague. This is an example of

  *A. irresponsible behavior.
   B. poor technical skill.
   C. illegal practice.
   D. communication error.

Reference: p. 241

Descriptors: 1. 15   2. 06   3. Interpretive
             4. 1 = No Process   5. Moderate

6. An example of accountable professional behavior would be

   A. performing CPR correctly.
  *B. providing medication for pain promptly.
   C. accurately reflecting upon a client's emotional needs.
   D. reviewing the pathophysiology of the client's medical diagnosis.

Reference: p. 241

Descriptors: 1. 15   2. 06   3. Interpretive
             4. 1 = No Process   5. Moderate

CHAPTER 16
Assessing

1. The purposes of the initial nursing assessment include all of the following except

   A. consideration of individual and family needs.
   B. examination of the client's ability to complete activities of daily living.
   C. provision of baseline information for the nursing record.
  *D. formulation of medical diagnoses.

Reference: pp. 248–249

Descriptors: 1. 16   2. 02, 03   3. Application
             4. 1 = No Process   5. Moderate

2. Which of the following is subjective client data?

   A. Drop in the client's blood pressure
  *B. Reported decrease in pain perception
   C. Ambulated without assistance in the hall this AM
   D. Sleeping quietly with eyes closed

Reference: pp. 248–250

Descriptors: 1. 16   2. 01, 04   3. Application
             4. 2 = Assessment   5. Moderate

3. A difference between nursing observation and interview is that

   A. observation provides only subjective data.
  *B. observation provides immediate data that can be subtantiated by the interview.
   C. interviews always glean more accurate data than observation.
   D. interviews take less time and energy.

Reference: pp. 249–250

Descriptors: 1. 16   2. 05   3. Application
             4. 1 = No Process   5. Easy

4. An appropriate introductory statement for the initial nursing interview is:

   A. "Hi, Sue! I'm John and I need you to answer these questions."
   B. "Please help me in completing this questionnaire, Ms. Jones."
   C. "My name is Jane, your nurse today. I'd like to get your history so I can plan your care."
  *D. "My name is J. Doe, your nurse today. May I ask you a few questions so we can plan your care together?"

Reference: pp. 250–252

Descriptors: 1. 16   2. 06   3. Application
             4. 1 = No Process   5. Moderate

5. Nursing assessment includes assessing all of the following except

   *A. the etiology of a client's disease.
   B. a client's ability to complete activities of daily living.
   C. a client's strengths and weaknesses.
   D. amount of data already collected.

   Reference: pp. 250–254

   Descriptors: 1. 16   2. 05   3. Application
                 4. 1 = No Process   5. Easy

6. Potential sources of client data necessary for a comprehensive assessment include all of the following except

   A. client.
   B. family.
   C. medical records.
   *D. sealed legal documents.

   Reference: p. 254

   Descriptors: 1. 16   2. 07   3. Factual
                 4. 1 = No Process   5. Easy

7. Differences between comprehensive and focused assessments include that

   A. subjective data are only included in the comprehensive assessment.
   B. focused assessments are not as important as comprehensive assessments.
   *C. focused assessments are usually ongoing, concerning specific problems.
   D. focused assessments cannot be a part of the initial assessment.

   Reference: p. 260

   Descriptors: 1. 16   2. 08   3. Interpretive
                 4. 2 = Assessment   5. Easy

8. Which of the following data is considered to be at the lowest priority to obtain when assessing a child with respiratory difficulties?

   A. Skin color
   *B. Dietary intake
   C. Vital signs
   D. Height and weight

   Reference: p. 262

   Descriptors: 1. 16   2. 09   3. Interpretive
                 4. 2 = Assessment   5. Difficult

9. Data that may need validation include

   A. confirmed reports when data are retrieved.
   *B. suspicious findings.
   C. supporting data for previous findings.
   D. client-reported findings.

   Reference: pp. 262–263

   Descriptors: 1. 16   2. 11   3. Application
                 4. 2 = Assessment   5. Easy

10. Which of the following findings is considered significant and requires immediate communication to the physician?

    A. Weight loss of 1 ounce in a 6 pound, 7 ounce infant
    *B. Diminished breath sounds in a client with pneumonia
    C. Change in blood pressure from 128/76 to 112/72
    D. Relief noted from prescribed pain medication

    Reference: pp. 263–264

    Descriptors: 1. 16   2. 12   3. Application
                  4. 3 = Analysis/Diag.   5. Difficult

CHAPTER 17
Diagnosing

1. Which of the following is a nursing diagnosis?

   A. Congestive heart failure
   *B. Anxiety
   C. Abnormal mammogram
   D. Impaired gas exchange, related to lung cancer

   Reference: pp. 267–268

   Descriptors: 1. 17   2. 01, 02   3. Interpretive
                 4. 3 = Analysis/Diag.   5. Moderate

2. A client undergoing surgery exhibits an elevated blood pressure of 188/112 and is pale and withdrawn. In order to understand the significance of this information, the nurse should first review the

   A. client's record for baseline vital signs.
   B. exisiting data to ascertain a pattern.
   C. medical record for orders for an anti-anxiety medication.
   *D. present client situation for more pertinent client data.

   Reference: pp. 272–273

   Descriptors: 1. 17   2. 01, 03   3. Application
                 4. 3 = Analysis/Diag.   5. Moderate

3. A healthy client who notes that his faith in God prevents him from seeking medical help has

   A. an actual client strength.
   B. a potential client strength.
   C. an actual client problem.
   *D. a potential client problem.

   Reference: p. 269

   Descriptors: 1. 17   2. 03   3. Interpretive
                 4. 3 = Analysis/Diag.   5. Moderate

4. A client states her faith prevents her from seeking medical assistance for actual health problems. An appropriate nursing response is to

   A. refer her to a psychologist.
   B. begin planning to assist her in overcoming her problem.
 *C. discuss with the client the potential problems that may occur without treatment.
   D. reinforce the client's spiritual awareness and present habits.

Reference: p. 269

Descriptors: 1. 17   2. 03   3. Application
             4. 5 = Implementation 5. Moderate

5. Which of the following statements is correct about this nursing diagnosis for a client on his way to surgery: "Actual mild anxiety related to impending surgery, as evidenced by the client's scared look and frightened appearance"?

   A. It is a medical diagnosis.
   B. The symptoms manifested are not related to the diagnosed problem.
 *C. This may not be a problem when considering the present situation.
   D. A scared look is too subjective to report.

Reference: pp. 270–273

Descriptors: 1. 17   2. 04   3. Interpretive
             4. 3 = Analysis/Diag. 5. Moderate

6. Advantages to using the NANDA-approved list of nursing diagnoses include

   A. promoting the use of an exclusive language among certain nursing specialties.
   B. allowing nurses to use computer-based programs.
   C. generating research for commonly used nursing interventions.
 *D. assisting in the organized nursing care of clients with similar illnesses.

Reference: p. 273

Descriptors: 1. 17   2. 07   3. Application
             4. 1 = No Process 5. Easy

7. Validation of derived nursing diagnoses can be done by which of the following methods?

 *A. Noting when a pattern emerges from the data retrieved
   B. Determining that the review of the data is not consistent with the defining characteristics of the diagnosis
   C. Being certain the diagnosis is amenable to medical care
   D. Asking three separate nurses to confirm the accuracy of the data

Reference: pp. 277–278

Descriptors: 1. 17   2. 05   3. Application
             4. 1 = No Process 5. Moderate

8. Utilizing Maslow's hierarchy of needs, which of the following nursing diagnoses has the highest priority?

   A. Severe anxiety, related to lifestyle changes
 *B. Ineffective breathing pattern
   C. Potential for injury
   D. Alteration in comfort

Reference: p. 278

Descriptors: 1. 17   2. 06   3. Application
             4. 4 = Planning   5. Moderate

9. A trauma victum is experiencing great pain. She is requesting that care be withheld until knowledge of her spouse's condition. The priority goal for planning nursing care is

   A. immediately relieving the client's pain.
   B. withholding all care until the condition of the client's spouse is known.
 *C. stabilizing the client's status while the spouse's condition is determined.
   D. having the client sign a consent for immediate surgery for self and spouse.

Reference: p. 278

Descriptors: 1. 17   2. 06   3. Interpretive
             4. 4 = Planning   5. Difficult

10. Ways to lessen the limitations of nursing diagnoses include

 *A. instituting great care in decreasing cultural misinterpretation.
   B. ensuring that the client is not involved in the planning process.
   C. utilizing the nursing diagnosis for medical concerns.
   D. using the same nursing diagnoses for all clients.

Reference: pp. 278–279

Descriptors: 1. 17   2. 07   3. Application
             4. 1 = No Process 5. Easy

CHAPTER 18
Planning

1. The most effective nursing plan of care to decrease postoperative abdominal pain includes

   A. teaching the client to use deep-breathing exercises.
   B. administering pain medications as ordered when needed.
   C. encouraging the client to ambulate 30 minutes prior to administering pain medication.
 *D. giving a back massage 30 minutes prior to the client's stated bedtime.

Reference: pp. 284–285

Descriptors: 1. 18   2. 01, 04 3. Application
             4. 5 = Implementation 5. Moderate

2. The most important purpose of planning care with the client is to

*A. individualize client care.
  B. assure continuity of care.
  C. use standardized care plans.
  D. provide a universal language for diagnosis.

Reference: p. 282

Descriptors: 1. 18   2. 02   3. Interpretive
             4. 1 = No Process   5. Moderate

3. The three basic elements to comprehensive planning include all of the following concepts except which?

  A. Planning is initially developed at time of admission.
  B. Plans are continuously updated.
  C. The discharge plan encompasses the client's needs for home care.
*D. Planning is solely a nursing activity.

Reference: pp. 283–284

Descriptors: 1. 18   2. 03   3. Interpretive
             4. 1 = No Process   5. Moderate

4. Of the following nursing actions, which would have the highest priority?

  A. Offer the client 60 cc juice between meals.
*B. Suction when signs and symptoms of dyspnea appear.
  C. Ambulate in hallway three times a day.
  D. Perform passive range of motion three times a day.

Reference: p. 284

Descriptors: 1. 18   2. 04   3. Interpretive
             4. 5 = Implementation 5. Moderate

5. An elderly diabetic client is hospitalized for pneumonia. A priority nursing diagnosis would be

*A. ineffective gas exchange.
  B. ineffective coping.
  C. potential for injury.
  D. nutritional alteration.

Reference: p. 284

Descriptors: 1. 18   2. 04   3. Interpretive
             4. 3 = Analysis/Diag.   5. Difficult

6. Which of the following is an example of a client goal for the nursing diagnosis "Alteration in comfort, related to surgery"?

  A. By the end of the shift, prescribed pain medication will be administered.
*B. By the end of the shift, the client will be able to do relaxation exercises.
  C. Before the end of the shift, the client will ambulate in the hallway.
  D. Before the end of the shift, teach the client deep breathing exercises.

Reference: pp. 291–296

Descriptors: 1. 18   2. 05, 06   3. Application
             4. 4 = Planning   5. Moderate

7. Which of the following is an example of a client goal for the nursing diagnosis "Severe anxiety related to impending surgery"?

  A. By the end of the shift, the client will receive anti-anxiety medication.
  B. By the end of the shift, discuss possible psychiatric consultation with physician.
*C. By the end of the shift, the client will experience a reduced level of anxiety.
  D. Administer medication as ordered throughout hospital stay.

Reference: pp. 291–296

Descriptors: 1. 18   2. 05, 06   3. Application
             4. 4 = Planning   5. Moderate

8. An appropriate nursing intervention for the diagnosis "Altered nutrition; less than body requirements" includes

*A. having the client keep a diet diary for three days.
  B. teaching the client to choose high-calorie snacks.
  C. advising the client to change culturally bound eating habits.
  D. encouraging the client to eat a high-protein diet.

Reference: p. 296

Descriptors: 1. 18   2. 06   3. Application
             4. 5 = Implementation 5. Moderate

9. When selecting appropriate nursing interventions, which of the following statements is true?

  A. Task-oriented interventions are best for client care.
  B. Communication skills are helpful only for psychological concerns.
*C. Individualization is necessary for optimal nursing care.
  D. It is rare that any one nursing intervention can solve a client's problem.

Reference: p. 296

Descriptors: 1. 18   2. 07   3. Interpretive
             4. 1 = No Process   5. Moderate

10. Possible remedies to decrease the problems related to the development of nursing care plans include all of the following except

  A. formation of an accurate, precise nursing diagnosis.
  B. goal development from a specific nursing diagnosis.
  C. maintenance of a current nursing care plan.
*D. utilizing only nurse-observed assessment data.

Reference: pp. 296–299

Descriptors: 1. 18   2. 08   3. Application
             4. 1 = No Process   5. Easy

CHAPTER 19
Implementing

1. The administration of prescribed pain medication is which type of nursing intervention?

   A. Independent
   *B. Dependent
   C. Interdependent
   D. Codependent

   Reference: p. 301

   Descriptors: 1. 19   2. 01, 02   3. Interpretive
              4. 1 = No Process   5. Easy

2. The withholding of a medication due to a severe allergic reaction is which type of nursing intervention?

   *A. Independent
   B. Dependent
   C. Interdependent
   D. Codependent

   Reference: p. 301

   Descriptors: 1. 19   2. 01, 02   3. Interpretive
              4. 1 = No Process   5. Moderate

3. Which of the following is not a prerequisite nursing skill necessary for implementing nursing orders?

   A. Intellectual
   B. Interpersonal
   C. Technical
   *D. Mechanical

   Reference: p. 308

   Descriptors: 1. 19   2. 04   3. Factual
              4. 1 = No Process   5. Easy

4. Critical thinking skills that assist the nurse in appropriately setting priorities are which type of nursing skill?

   *A. Intellectual
   B. Interpersonal
   C. Technical
   D. Mechanical

   Reference: p. 308

   Descriptors: 1. 19   2. 05   3. Application
              4. 1 = No Process   5. Easy

5. Variables that influence the implementation of nursing interventions include all of the following except

   *A. consideration of the client's stated religion.
   B. the nurse's expectations of self-performance.
   C. nursing unit staffing.
   D. the physician's competencies.

   Reference: pp. 307–310

   Descriptors: 1. 19   2. 05   3. Application
              4. 1 = No Process   5. Easy

6. To develop skill in implementing nursing interventions, the nurse should

   A. admit to the client the nurse's uncertainty prior to completion of a new skill.
   *B. develop a varied repertoire of skills and techniques gleaned from peers.
   C. utilize random nursing interventions until one works.
   D. use only interventions that are procedure-based.

   Reference: p. 302

   Descriptors: 1. 19   2. 06   3. Application
              4. 1 = No Process   5. Easy

7. The primary purpose of ongoing data collection in care planning is to

   A. determine if a previous nursing measure solved the problem.
   *B. review the care plan and update as necessary.
   C. develop a comprehensive data base.
   D. ensure data collection from all relevant sources.

   Reference: p. 311

   Descriptors: 1. 19   2. 07   3. Application
              4. 1 = No Process   5. Easy

CHAPTER 20
Evaluating

1. In the evaluation step of the nursing process, the nurse decides whether the goal

   *A. has been achieved.
   B. has been set.
   C. is mutually derived.
   D. was appropriate for the medical diagnosis.

   Reference: p. 314

   Descriptors: 1. 20   2. 01, 02   3. Factual
              4. 1 = No Process   5. Easy

2. The evaluation step of the nursing process

   A. may reveal a "new" client condition.
   *B. reflects only the nurse's judgment about the client's response to mutually set goals.
   C. is completed only by the client.
   D. is the end phase of a static process.

   Reference: pp. 314–315

   Descriptors: 1. 20   2. 02   3. Application
              4. 1 = No Process   5. Easy

3. Evaluation of client goal achievement includes all of the following except

   A. physical changes.
   B. time criteria.
   C. skill attainment.
   *D. intervention completion.

   Reference: pp. 315–316

   Descriptors: 1. 20   2. 02, 03   3. Factual
              4. 1 = No Process   5. Easy

4. A successful resolution of the nursing goal "By the end of the shift, the client will state a reduction in postoperative pain to a 2/10 level" is if

A. pain medication was received twice during the shift.
*B. client stated pain relief at 10 PM on 1/10 scale.
C. client is able to ambulate in the hallway.
D. client is talking freely.

Reference: pp. 319–322

Descriptors: 1. 20   2. 03   3. Interpretive
4. 6 = Evaluation   5. Moderate

5. Factors that influence goal achievement include the

*A. client's age and developmental goals.
B. nurse's ability to focus on the client.
C. strong commitment by the institution to client care.
D. nurse's commitment to the utilization of the nursing process.

Reference: pp. 319–322

Descriptors: 1. 20   2. 04   3. Application
4. 1 = No Process   5. Moderate

6. An obese client did not meet the goal "By the end of the second week, the client will be able to follow a 1500-calorie reduction diet." The nurse and client should reassess the

A. client's actual weight.
*B. client's ability to maintain a 1500-calorie diet.
C. nurse's feelings about obese clients.
D. health care agency's ability to provide the prescribed diet.

Reference: pp. 319–322

Descriptors: 1. 20   2. 04, 05   3. Interpretive
4. 6 = Evaluation   5. Moderate

7. A client has an order for Demerol 100 mg every 4 hours as needed for pain relief. The nurse has been giving the medication every 4 hours, but notes the pain medication is unsuccessful in relieving the client's pain. Revision of the nursing care plan can include

A. giving the pain medication more frequently.
B. increasing the dosage of the pain medication.
*C. teaching the client deep breathing and relaxation exercises.
D. explaining that postoperative pain is temporary.

Reference: pp. 319–322

Descriptors: 1. 20   2. 05   3. Application
4. 6 = Evaluation   5. Moderate

8. A diabetic client is unable to draw up the insulin into the syringe by the mutually set time. Revision of the nursing care plan includes

A. ordering an eye exam for the client.
*B. assessing the client's visual acuity.
C. ordering an in-depth learning assessment.
D. reviewing the client's need for insulin and prescribing a new medication.

Reference: pp. 319–322

Descriptors: 1. 20   2. 05   3. Application
4. 6 = Evaluation   5. Moderate

9. Quality assurance programs assist nursing in providing effective health care in that they

*A. enable the profession to be accountable to society.
B. identify values and standards inherent to medicine.
C. establish criteria that recommend punishment if deficiencies are noted.
D. help contain health care costs.

Reference: pp. 322–324

Descriptors: 1. 20   2. 06   3. Factual
4. 1 = No Process   5. Easy

10. Strategies to assist the nurse in self-evaluation include all of the following except

A. journal-keeping of professional experiences and reactions.
B. nursing symposia to discuss care delivery situations.
C. identification of master nurses and implementation of a mentoring system.
*D. public reporting of medication errors.

Reference: pp. 324–326

Descriptors: 1. 20   2. 07   3. Application
4. 1 = No Process   5. Moderate

CHAPTER 21
Documenting, Reporting, and Conferring

1. Which of the following statements denotes understanding of guidelines for effective documentation?

A. "I can erase mistakes or errors as needed."
B. "It's okay to chart another nurse's interventions as my own."
*C. "Usage of scales or ratios for pain management is appropriate."
D. "Once I sign the narrative notes, I don't have to sign subsequent entries."

Reference: pp. 330–332

Descriptors: 1. 21   2. 02   3. Interpretive
4. 1 = No Process   5. Moderate

2. The nurse gathers the following client assessment data: decreased swelling in both legs, from a 4/5 to a 2/5 scale; skin feels warm and dry, pink in color. Appropriate documentation is

   *A. "Bilateral edema decreased from 4/5 to 2/5 scale."
   B. "Skin color WNL."
   C. "Swelling in both legs down decreased."
   D. "Skin color and circulation improved from previous assessment."

   Reference: pp. 330–332

   Descriptors: 1. 21   2. 02   3. Application
                4. 2 = Assessment   5. Moderate

3. Which of the following is not a purpose of client records? To

   A. evaluate effectiveness of nursing interventions.
   B. increase understanding of nursing regimen.
   C. portray client's condition.
   *D. judge client's worthiness for health care.

   Reference: p. 333

   Descriptors: 1. 21   2. 04   3. Application
                4. 1 = No Process   5. Moderate

4. An appropriate method of documentation for critically ill clients with multiple problems requiring a highly individualized care plan is

   A. the case management model.
   B. PIE format.
   C. charting by exception.
   *D. SOAP notes.

   Reference: pp. 333–337

   Descriptors: 1. 21   2. 05   3. Interpretive
                4. 1 = No Process   5. Moderate

5. Physicians' records, nurses' notes, graphic sheets, and diagnostic records describe which method of documentation?

   *A. Source-oriented medical records
   B. Problem-oriented records
   C. Case-management records
   D. Focus-charting records

   Reference: pp. 333–334

   Descriptors: 1. 21   2. 05   3. Application
                4. 1 = No Process   5. Moderate

6. The client's skin condition upon admission is typically found on which documentation form?

   *A. Initial nursing assessment
   B. Nursing care plan
   C. Graphic record
   D. Progress notes

   Reference: p. 337

   Descriptors: 1. 21   2. 06   3. Application
                4. 1 = No Process   5. Moderate

7. A summary of the client's condition upon discharge from an institution is found on which documentation form?

   A. Initial nursing assessment
   B. Nursing care plan
   C. Home care documentation
   *D. Discharge summary

   Reference: pp. 337–339

   Descriptors: 1. 21   2. 06   3. Application
                4. 1 = No Process   5. Moderate

8. Charting practices that create potential legal problems include all of the following except

   A. inconsistent data and times listed.
   B. use of correction fluid and erasers.
   C. vague or discrepant assessment data.
   *D. accurate, holistic data noted.

   Reference: pp. 339–342

   Descriptors: 1. 21   2. 07   3. Application
                4. 1 = No Process   5. Moderate

9. Which of the following nursing documentation entries reflects a potential legal risk?

   A. "Skin pink, warm, dry over bilateral lower extremities."
   *B. "Client smelled bad and has substandard hygiene practices."
   C. "Client states is happy going home today."
   D. "Client ambulated without difficulty in hallway with 1 assist."

   Reference: p. 339

   Descriptors: 1. 21   2. 07   3. Interpretive
                4. 1 = No Process   5. Moderate

10. It is 3 AM. The nurse assesses a critical change in a client's condition. Which of the following modes of communication is most appropriate?

    A. Written report
    B. Change of shift report
    *C. Telephone report
    D. Computer message

    Reference: pp. 340–341

    Descriptors: 1. 21   2. 08   3. Interpretive
                 4. 5 = Implementation 5. Moderate

CHAPTER 22
Communicator

1. In effective communication, the source sends a message to the receiver. Which of the following describes the process by which reception and comprehension of the message are verified?

   A. Noise
   *B. Feedback
   C. Channel
   D. Decoder

   Reference: pp. 359, 360

   Descriptors: 1. 22   2. 01, 02   3. Factual
            4. 1 = No Process 5. Easy

2. Forms of nonverbal communication include

   A. sleeping.
   B. facing the client while speaking.
   *C. posturing.
   D. conversing on the telephone.

   Reference: pp. 360–362

   Descriptors: 1. 22   2. 03   3. Factual
            4. 1 = No Process 5. Easy

3. Effective interviewing skills are important to the nursing process because

   *A. they elicit accurate, comprehensive information for assessments.
   B. accurate evaluation depends on correctly interpreting only verbal cues.
   C. data for physical assessment can only be obtained through an interview.
   D. interviews are the only way information can be received about the client.

   Reference: pp. 364–366

   Descriptors: 1. 22   2. 04   3. Application
            4. 1 = No Process 5. Moderate

4. Appropriate client goals for the orientation phase of the helping relationship include

   A. evaluating the relationship between the participants.
   *B. completing the clarification of the caregiver/care recipient roles.
   C. introducing the caregivers to the care recipients.
   D. assisting the care recipient in receiving care.

   Reference: pp. 367–368

   Descriptors: 1. 22   2. 05   3. Application
            4. 4 = Planning 5. Moderate

5. An appropriate client goal when in the working phase of the helping relationship is to

   A. know the names of the health care providers.
   *B. demonstrate cast care.
   C. know when meal times occur.
   D. evaluate the effectiveness of the relationship.

   Reference: pp. 367–368

   Descriptors: 1. 22   2. 05   3. Application
            4. 4 = Planning 5. Moderate

6. Successful resolution of a helping relationship includes the following characteristic:

   A. established mutual agreement on the duration of the relationship.
   B. cooperation in goal-directed activities.
   C. free expression of feelings about the health care provider.
   *D. identification of progress towards the mutually set goals.

   Reference: pp. 367–368

   Descriptors: 1. 22   2. 05   3. Application
            4. 6 = Evaluation 5. Moderate

7. A client with whom the nurse has established a positive relationship is apparently agitated. When asked if anything is wrong, the client states anxiously, "Oh, nothing, not really." The nurse should

   *A. sit beside the client and wait a few minutes in silence.
   B. leave the room to return later.
   C. tell the client, "Okay," and discuss another matter.
   D. express feelings of being hurt and rejected.

   Reference: pp. 369–371

   Descriptors: 1. 22   2. 06   3. Application
            4. 5 = Implementation 5. Moderate

8. A Hispanic client is admitted to the unit. The nurse states, "I can't speak Spanish, so I can't help her." This is an example of

   A. caring.
   B. logical thinking.
   *C. prejudice.
   D. concern.

   Reference: pp. 369–371

   Descriptors: 1. 22   2. 08   3. Application
            4. 1 = No Process 5. Moderate

9. A client with AIDS who is a nurse tells the visitor, "I wish I would've told them that I was a nurse because I would have gotten better care." This is an example of

*A. stereotyping due to the client's occupation.
B. avoidance of the client's teaching needs.
C. stereotyping due to the client's condition.
D. nonassertiveness on the client's part.

Reference: pp. 369–371

Descriptors: 1. 22   2. 08   3. Application
            4. 1 = No Process   5. Moderate

10. The most effective way to communicate with the hard of hearing is to

A. raise the voice.
*B. sit directly in front of the client.
C. increase the lighting in the client's room.
D. exaggerate mouth movements so the client can read the nurse's lips.

Reference: pp. 371–373

Descriptors: 1. 22   2. 09   3. Application
            4. 5 = Implementation 5. Moderate

11. Nursing guidelines when caring for a client from a different culture should include

A. assuming the client's background is similiar to the nurse.
B. refering all clients to an interpreter prior to providing care.
C. assuming the client understands traditional medical practices.
*D. validating understanding to avoid misunderstanding.

Reference: p. 376

Descriptors: 1. 22   2. 06   3. Application
            4. 5 = Implementation 5. Moderate

12. Characteristics of an effective group process include all of the following except that

A. all group members possess mutual trust.
*B. personal goals are more important than group goals.
C. a strong sense of commitment is felt among group members.
D. aims and goals are clearly understood by all group members.

Reference: pp. 382–383

Descriptors: 1. 22   2. 10   3. Interpretive
            4. 1 = No Process   5. Moderate

CHAPTER 23
Teacher and Counselor

1. An example of cognitive learning is a/an

A. demonstration of correct injection technique.
*B. successful completion of a test on diabetes pathophysiology.
C. understanding of one's anger over having diabetes.
D. expression of excitement over learning how to self-inject.

Reference: p. 388

Descriptors: 1. 23   2. 01, 02 3. Application
            4. 1 = No Process   5. Moderate

2. Which of the following clients has the developmental maturity to self-catheterize?

A. A 16-year-old with a fractured dominant arm
*B. A 10-year-old with full range of motion in both hands
C. A severely mentally retarded 12-year-old with normal motor skills
D. A healthy 12-year-old with hemiplegia

Reference: pp. 388–389

Descriptors: 1. 23   2. 02   3. Interpretive
            4. 3 = Analysis/Diag. 5. Moderate

3. The primary consideration in increasing the effectiveness of teaching a client how to care for a colostomy is to

A. use a videotaped demonstration.
B. use written materials with diagrams.
*C. assess the client's readiness to learn.
D. encourage the client to immediately begin to do self-care.

Reference: pp. 388–389

Descriptors: 1. 23   2. 03   3. Application
            4. 2 = Assessment   5. Moderate

4. A primipara is having difficulty in diapering her newborn and is repeatedly asking how to care for the circumcision site. An appropriate nursing diagnosis is

A. knowledge deficit: infant care, related to inexperience.
B. potential for infection: infant care, related to inexperience.
*C. potential altered parenting: infant care, related to inexperience and anxiety.
D. ineffective coping: infant care, related to a new role.

Reference: p. 393

Descriptors: 1. 23   2. 04   3. Interpretive
            4. 3 = Analysis/Diag. 5. Difficult

5. A teaching care plan for a 10-year-old insulin-dependent diabetic should include

   A. teaching the client how to weigh his own food.
   B. showing the client a comic book about children with diabetes.
   *C. assessing his ability to hold a pencil and manipulate a syringe.
   D. first teaching his parents about his particular needs.

   Reference: pp. 393–398

   Descriptors: 1. 23   2. 05, 02   3. Application
                4. 5 = Implementation 5. Moderate

6. Consideration in implementing a low-impact exercise program for an elderly client with rheumatoid arthritis includes

   *A. easy first-floor access.
   B. dim lighting to decrease eye strain.
   C. use of music to maintain aerobic pace.
   D. weight-lifting equipment to increase strength.

   Reference: pp. 393–398

   Descriptors: 1. 23   2. 02, 05   3. Application
                4. 5 = Implementation 5. Moderate

7. Considerations in implementing infant day care for health care workers include

   A. providing pull toys and small, button-like toys for play.
   *B. working hours for weekend and night coverage.
   C. providing play pens for sleeping in groups.
   D. purchasing finger foods for oral satisfaction.

   Reference: pp. 393–398

   Descriptors: 1. 23   2. 02, 05   3. Application
                4. 5 = Implementation 5. Moderate

8. The best method to evaluate a client's ability to change a dressing includes

   A. having the client orally describe how to change to dressing.
   *B. having the client change the dressing with the nurse observing.
   C. gauging the client's reaction while the nurse changes the dressing.
   D. having the client complete and pass a written exam on how to change a dressing.

   Reference: p. 402

   Descriptors: 1. 23   2. 06   3. Application
                4. 6 = Evaluation   5. Moderate

9. Counseling includes all of the following interpersonal skills except

   A. listening.
   *B. advising.
   C. providing suggestions.
   D. using problem-solving skills.

   Reference: p. 404

   Descriptors: 1. 23   2. 01, 10   3. Factual
                4. 1 = No Process   5. Easy

10. The relationship between the nursing process and problem-solving process is that the nursing process is

    A. a formal method of problem-solving.
    B. limited in its ability to problem-solve.
    *C. a problem-solving technique.
    D. focused on client outcomes.

    Reference: p. 408

    Descriptors: 1. 23   2. 09   3. Application
                 4. 1 = No Process   5. Moderate

11. The nurse demonstrated crutch walking for a client, and the client returned the demonstration. Appropriate documentation includes

    A. "Crutch walking teaching done."
    B. "Client given crutch walking demonstration."
    C. "Client demonstrated appropriate crutch walking."
    *D. "Crutch walking demonstration given with appropriate client return demonstration."

    Reference: p. 404

    Descriptors: 1. 23   2. 07   3. Interpretive
                 4. 5 = Implementation 5. Moderate

12. A teenage client who is experiencing depression and suicidal tendencies is admitted to the hospital. An appropriate form of counseling would include

    A. intensive short-term counseling.
    B. long-term weekly counseling.
    *C. intensive short-term and long-term counseling.
    D. motivational counseling to complete rehabilitation.

    Reference: pp. 407–409

    Descriptors: 1. 23   2. 10   3. Interpretive
                 4. 5 = Implementation 5. Moderate

CHAPTER 24
Leader, Researcher, and Advocate

1. Leadership skills necessary for staff nurses include all of the following except

   A. ability to establish positive professional roles with clients and peers.
   B. critical thinking skills to problem solve.
   C. organizational skills to improve time management.
   *D. ability to criticize and critique a peer's performance.

   Reference: pp. 412, 414

   Descriptors: 1. 24   2. 02, 05   3. Application
                4. 1 = No Process   5. Easy

2. The difference between a mentorship and a preceptorship is that

  A. mentors provide advice and assistance to the protégé.
  *B. preceptors are paid employees of the hiring institution.
  C. preceptors assist the orientee in informal networking.
  D. selection of a mentor is done by administration.

Reference: pp. 420, 421

Descriptors: 1. 24   2. 01, 05   3. Application
            4. 1 = No Process   5. Moderate

3. Basic research skills that nurses in a caregiver role utilize include

  A. isolation of research findings from practice areas.
  *B. questioning current care practices and rationale.
  C. advising clients to participate in research.
  D. changing medical treatments as part of research.

Reference: pp. 421–422

Descriptors: 1. 24   2. 07   3. Application
            4. 1 = No Process   5. Easy

4. The family of a patient who is dying asks about the possibility of organ donation and requests information. The nurse should

  A. provide them with a lawyer.
  B. ask the family to wait to discuss donation until after the client is deceased.
  *C. contact the physician concerning the family's concerns and wishes.
  D. tell the family that they should contact their clergy for advice.

Reference: pp. 424–427

Descriptors: 1. 24   2. 09, 10   3. Application
            4. 5 = Implementation   5. Moderate

5. The nurse knows the client understands living wills and advanced directives when he

  *A. decides what type of care he wishes to receive in special circumstances.
  B. wants his family to make the decision.
  C. repeatedly asks for advice.
  D. states the decision is irreversible.

Reference: pp. 424–427

Descriptors: 1. 24   2. 10   3. Interpretive
            4. 6 = Evaluation   5. Moderate

6. Revising a catheter change routine due to a recent research finding is an example of which knowledge source?

  *A. Scientific
  B. Authoritative
  C. Traditional
  D. Personal

Reference: pp. 422–423

Descriptors: 1. 24   2. 06   3. Application
            4. 1 = No Process   5. Easy

7. The charge nurse calls a meeting to discuss the recent staffing shortage. The staff devises a short-term and a long-term proposal to solve the problem. This is an example of which type of leadership?

  A. Autocratic
  *B. Democratic
  C. Laissez-faire
  D. Transformational

Reference: pp. 414–416

Descriptors: 1. 24   2. 02   3. Interpretive
            4. 1 = No Process   5. Easy

8. A client expresses concerns over upcoming surgery. The first nursing response would be to

  A. document the client's concerns.
  B. persuade the client to continue with the surgery.
  *C. further explore the client's feelings.
  D. cancel the surgery.

Reference: pp. 425–426

Descriptors: 1. 24   2. 09   3. Application
            4. 5 = Implementation 5. Difficult

9. An example of ineffective nursing management on a busy surgical unit would be

  A. increasing staff numbers when the surgery schedule is the heaviest.
  B. engaging the staff in new equipment purchases.
  C. providing staff development on the latest research findings.
  *D. maintaining the status quo regardless of health care changes.

Reference: p. 416

Descriptors: 1. 24   2. 03   3. Interpretive
            4. 5 = Implementation 5. Moderate

10. New graduates typically engage in all of the following areas of leadership except

  A. providing guidance to clients.
  *B. assuming full-time managerial positions.
  C. upholding institutional policies and regulations.
  D. participating in clinically based research.

Reference: pp. 419–420

Descriptors: 1. 24   2. 05   3. Interpretive
            4. 1 = No Process   5. Easy

UNIT VI
ACTIONS BASIC TO NURSING CARE

CHAPTER 25
Vital Signs

1. A 76-year-old client hospitalized following abdominal surgery has a temperature of 38°C (100.4°F). The nurse plans to assess the client's vital signs every

    A. 30 minutes.
    B. 60 minutes.
    *C. 4 hours.
    D. 8 hours.

    Reference: p. 433

    Descriptors: 1. 25   2. 02   3. Application
                 4. 4 = Planning   5. Easy

2. The nurse plans to assess an adult client's core body temperature. The nurse should explain to the client that her temperature will be measured using which of the following sites?

    A. Axillary
    B. Popliteal
    C. Oral
    *D. Rectal

    Reference: p. 434

    Descriptors: 1. 25   2. 02   3. Application
                 4. 5 = Implementation 5. Moderate

3. The nurse explains to an adult client who is shivering that shivering is a response that increases the production of heat and is initiated by the body's

    *A. hypothalamus.
    B. pituitary.
    C. thyroid.
    D. thalamus.

    Reference: p. 434

    Descriptors: 1. 25   2. 01   3. Factual
                 4. 5 = Implementation 5. Easy

4. At 5 PM the nurse determines that a 25-year-old client has an oral temperature of 37.5°C (99.5°F) 8 hours after an appendectomy. The nurse should

    A. immediately contact the client's physician.
    B. offer the client ice water to reduce the fever.
    C. increase the intravenous fluid rate.
    *D. continue to monitor the client's vital signs.

    Reference: pp. 434, 437

    Descriptors: 1. 25   2. 02   3. Application
                 4. 5 = Implementation 5. Moderate

5. A client is admitted to the hospital from the emergency room with a temperature of 105.8°F. The nurse determines that the client is experiencing

    *A. hyperpyrexia.
    B. hypopyrexia.
    C. hyperemia.
    D. hypothermia.

    Reference: p. 435

    Descriptors: 1. 25   2. 01   3. Factual
                 4. 3 = Analysis/Diag.   5. Easy

6. The emergency room nurse examines an adult client who has intense shivering, rigid muscles, dilated pupils, and bluish skin. The nurse determines that the client is most likely experiencing

    *A. hypothermia.
    B. hyperthermia.
    C. circulatory collapse.
    D. shock.

    Reference: p. 436

    Descriptors: 1. 25   2. 02   3. Interpretive
                 4. 3 = Analysis/Diag.   5. Moderate

7. An adult client visits the emergency room after playing tennis on a hot summer day. He complains of fatigue and nausea and his skin is moist. The client's oral temperature is 37.8°C (100°F). The nurse determines that the client is most likely experiencing heat

    A. cramps.
    *B. exhaustion.
    C. syncope.
    D. stroke.

    Reference: p. 436

    Descriptors: 1. 25   2. 01   3. Interpretive
                 4. 3 = Analysis/Diag.   5. Moderate

8. The nurse is preparing to assess an adult client's oral temperature using an electronic thermometer. The nurse explains the procedure to the client and determines that the client understands the instructions when the client says electronic thermometers

    *A. measure body temperature in 25 to 30 seconds.
    B. are less accurate when used with children.
    C. reduce infection because all of the equipment is disposable.
    D. are usually more accurate than glass thermometers.

    Reference: pp. 437–438

    Descriptors: 1. 25   2. 03   3. Application
                 4. 6 = Evaluation   5. Moderate

9. The nurse instructs the mother of a 2-week-old infant about checking her child's temperature. The nurse determines that the mother needs *further* instructions when she says,

   A. "I should check the temperature using the axillary site."
   B. "A glass thermometer should be left in place for at least 3 minutes."
   C. "A digital thermometer can determine the temperature quickly."
  *D. "I can use a tympanic membrane device to check the temperature."

Reference: p. 437

Descriptors: 1. 25   2. 06   3. Application
             4. 6 = Evaluation   5. Moderate

10. After assessing an adult client's rectal temperature, the nurse documents both the temperature and the site in the client's record since

  *A. different readings will be obtained from each site.
   B. diarrhea is common following a rectal temperature.
   C. infections can influence the temperature at each site.
   D. the oral route is the most commonly used site.

Reference: pp. 437, 439

Descriptors: 1. 25   2. 03   3. Application
             4. 5 = Implementaion 5. Moderate

11. The nurse is caring for several clients on a surgical unit of a hospital. The nurse should assess a client's temperature using the rectal site if the client is

  *A. receiving oxygen by mask.
   B. receiving oxygen by nasal cannula.
   C. recovering from cardiac surgery.
   D. unable to speak clearly.

Reference: p. 439

Descriptors: 1. 25   2. 02   3. Application
             4. 2 = Assessment   5. Moderate

12. The nurse has instructed a client about taking her 4-year-old child's temperature. The nurse determines that the client needs *further* instructions when she says,

  *A. "The preferred site for children is the oral route."
   B. "I shouldn't use the oral route with a glass thermometer."
   C. "I should wash my hands before taking my child's temperature."
   D. "The tympanic membrane temperature is a core body temperature."

Reference: pp. 441, 445

Descriptors: 1. 25   2. 06   3. Interpretive
             4. 6 = Evaluation   5. Moderate

13. The nurse is planning to instruct a client about taking her father's temperature at home. Which of the following would be important to include in the teaching plan?

   A. Wash a glass thermometer after use with hot, soapy water.
   B. Place a glass thermometer under the tongue for 5 minutes.
   C. Shake the thermometer before use to 98.6°F.
  *D. Wait at least 30 minutes after eating before taking the client's temperature.

References: pp. 441, 448

Descriptors: 1. 25   2. 06   3. Application
             4. 4 = Planning   5. Moderate

14. Four hours after knee surgery, a 78-year-old client has a pulse rate of 110 beats per minute. The nurse should assess the client for

   A. increased blood pressure.
   B. hypothermia.
  *C. pain.
   D. dysrhythmia.

Reference: p. 446

Descriptors: 1. 25   2. 02   3. Application
             4. 2 = Assessment   5. Easy

15. Before obtaining an axillary temperature of an adult client with a glass thermometer, the nurse explains to the client that the

   A. thermometer will remain in place for 5 minutes.
   B. axillary temperature is 1° higher than the rectal temperature.
   C. method is not used with children under 6 years of age.
  *D. deepest area of the axilla provides the most accuracy.

Reference: p. 447

Descriptors: 1. 25   2. 05   3. Application
             4. 5 = Implementation 5. Moderate

16. The nurse notifies the physician when it is determined that an adult male client's pulse is 52 beats per minute because the client is experiencing

   A. cardiovascular collapse.
  *B. bradycardia.
   C. tachycardia.
   D. dysrhythmia.

Reference: p. 448

Descriptors: 1. 25   2. 03   3. Interpretive
             4. 3 = Analysis/Diag. 5. Easy

17. The nurse is preparing an adult client for an electrocardiogram. The nurse plans to position the client for electrode placement by placing the client in a

A. prone position.
B. side-lying position.
*C. supine position.
D. Trendelenburg position.

Reference: p. 449

Descriptors: 1. 25   2. 05   3. Application
          4. 4 = Planning   5. Easy

18. To assess pulse deficit of an adult client, the nurse taking the apical pulse plans to

A. place the stethoscope at the client's third intercostal space.
B. place the client in a side-lying position.
*C. ask another nurse to assist with the procedure.
D. ask the client to take a deep breath.

Reference: p. 452

Descriptors: 1. 25   2. 05   3. Application
          4. 4 = Planning   5. Easy

19. A mother of a 4-year-old child tells the nurse that she is worried because the child holds her breath during temper tantrums and turns red in the face. The nurse should instruct the mother that

A. excessive carbon monoxide can cause brain damage.
B. the family needs intensive counseling.
C. unconsciousness can occur as a result of this behavior.
*D. chemical stimulation of the respiratory center will eventually cause breathing.

Reference: p. 456

Descriptors: 1. 25   2. 06   3. Application
          4. 5 = Implementation 5. Moderate

20. The nurse notes that a hospitalized adult client has orthopnea. The nurse plans to assess the client's respirations while the client

A. lies in a side-lying position in bed.
*B. sits upright in a chair.
C. has the head of the bed elevated 20°.
D. lies supine in bed.

Reference: p. 456

Descriptors: 1. 25   2. 02   3. Application
          4. 4 = Planning   5. Easy

21. The nurse is assessing a 2-year-old hospitalized with a respiratory infection. The nurse determines that the client's breath sounds indicate a harsh, high-pitched sound on inspiration. The nurse documents the client's

A. gurgles.
B. wheezes.
C. crackles.
*D. stridor.

Reference: p. 456

Descriptors: 1. 25   2. 01   3. Interpretive
          4. 3 = Analysis/Diag.   5. Moderate

22. The nurse assesses an elderly client with terminal cancer and determines that the client's respirations gradually increase, then decrease, and then there is a period of apnea. The nurse determines that the client is experiencing respirations termed

*A. Cheyne-Stokes.
B. Biot's.
C. bradypnea.
D. eupnea.

Reference: p. 458

Descriptors: 1. 25   2. 02   3. Factual
          4. 3 = Analysis/Diag.   5. Easy

23. The nurse is caring for a client who was admitted to the hospital following a severe automobile accident. The client's respirations are 14 per minute, shallow, and irregular. The nurse plans to monitor the client for possible

A. infection.
B. abdominal injury.
*C. head injury.
D. hypertension.

Reference: p. 456

Descriptors: 1. 25   2. 02   3. Interpretive
          4. 4 = Planning   5. Moderate

24. An adult client received a dose of meperidine hydrochloride (Demerol) 30 minutes ago. Before ambulation, the nurse should assess the client for

A. tachycardia.
B. hypertension.
*C. hypotension.
D. tachypnea.

Reference: p. 460

Descriptors: 1. 25   2. 01   3. Application
          4. 2 = Assessment   5. Moderate

25. The nurse determines pulse pressure of a client by

   A. subtracting the pulse rate from the systolic pressure.
   *B. subtracting the diastolic reading from the systolic reading.
   C. determining the amount of pressure required for the apical pulse.
   D. determining the difference between the apical and radial pulses.

   Reference: p. 457

   Descriptors: 1. 25   2. 01   3. Application
                4. 5 = Implementation 5. Moderate

26. The nurse has instructed a group of adults at a local senior citizens center about blood pressure and hypertension. The nurse determines that one of the members of the group understands the instructions when she says,

   *A. "Blood pressure increases as one ages due to decreased elasticity of the arteries."
   B. "Women usually have a higher blood pressure than men."
   C. "Blood pressure is lowest during the late afternoon."
   D. "After eating, blood pressure usually falls, then rises before sleep."

   Reference: p. 458

   Descriptors: 1. 25   2. 06   3. Application
                4. 6 = Evaluation   5. Moderate

27. The nurse is preparing to assist a client to ambulate for the first time after a period of bedrest following gall bladder surgery. Before ambulation, the nurse should assess the client for

   A. decreased respiratory rate.
   B. increased pulse pressure.
   *C. orthostatic hypotension.
   D. secondary hypertension.

   Reference: p. 459

   Descriptors: 1. 25   2. 03   3. Application
                4. 2 = Assessment   5. Easy

28. The nurse is preparing to assess a client's blood pressure. In order to identify the first Korotkoff sound accurately, the nurse should

   A. place the cuff about 3 inches above the elbow.
   B. reinflate the cuff once air is released to recheck rate.
   C. repeat any suspicious reading within 10 seconds.
   *D. inflate the cuff while palpating the artery and note the reading where the pulse disappears.

   Reference: p. 464

   Descriptors: 1. 25   2. 02   3. Application
                4. 5 = Implementation 5. Moderate

29. A client diagnosed with hypertension asks the nurse about blood pressure monitoring equipment for home use. The nurse should instruct the client that

   A. digital blood pressure monitoring equipment is not very accurate.
   B. if there is difficulty hearing the blood pressure sounds, lower the arm for 15 seconds.
   C. home monitoring of a client's blood pressure is not recommended.
   *D. cuff sizes vary and a poorly fitting cuff can produce an inaccurate measurement.

   Reference: p. 466

   Descriptors: 1. 25   2. 06   3. Application
                4. 5 = Implementation 5. Moderate

30. The nurse has instructed an adult client how to monitor her blood pressure while at home. The nurse determines that the client has understood the instructions when the client says,

   *A. "A cuff that is too small will result in falsely high readings."
   B. "I can record the systolic and diastolic measurement by the sensory detection method."
   C. "Misplacing the bell beyond the direct area of the artery can result in falsely high readings."
   D. "Monitoring my blood pressure at home means that I don't need to have it checked periodically by a nurse."

   Reference: p. 467

   Descriptors: 1. 25   2. 06   3. Application
                4. 6 = Evaluation   5. Moderate

CHAPTER 26
Health Assessment

1. A major purpose of a health assessment of an adult client is to

   A. identify client weaknesses.
   B. establish client confidence.
   C. evaluate the effects of aging.
   *D. establish a nurse-client relationship.

   Reference: p. 474

   Descriptors: 1. 26   2. 02   3. Factual
                4. 1 = No Process   5. Easy

2. The nurse is planning to examine an adult client's internal eye structures. The nurse should explain to the client that the purpose of the numbers on the rotating dial of the ophthalmoscope is to

   A. control illumination of the lens.
   *B. adjust magnification power of the lens.
   C. determine visual acuity.
   D. test extraocular movements.

   Reference: p. 474

   Descriptors: 1. 26   2. 04   3. Application
                4. 5 = Implementation 5. Moderate

3. In order to examine a client's external ear canal and tympanic membrane, the nurse plans to use a/an

   A. tuning fork.
   B. Snellen chart.
   C. inspection probe.
   *D. otoscope.

   Reference: p. 475

   Descriptors: 1. 26   2. 05   3. Application
                4. 4 = Planning   5. Easy

4. To assess full lung expansion of an adult client, the nurse plans to place the client in which position?

   A. Supine
   B. Side-lying
   C. Trendelenburg
   *D. Sitting

   Reference: p. 476

   Descriptors: 1. 26   2. 06   3. Application
                4. 4 = Planning   5. Moderate

5. To assess an adult client's abdomen and peripheral pulses, the nurse begins by placing the client in a

   *A. supine position.
   B. lithotomy position.
   C. Sim's position.
   D. sitting position.

   Reference: p. 476

   Descriptors: 1. 26   2. 06   3. Application
                4. 5 = Implementation 5. Moderate

6. The nurse is planning to perform a physical assessment on an adult client. Before the examination, the nurse should ask the client to

   A. remove all jewelry.
   *B. empty the bladder.
   C. have a bowel movement.
   D. take several deep breaths.

   Reference: p. 478

   Descriptors: 1. 26   2. 04   3. Application
                4. 5 = Implementation 5. Moderate

7. During a physical examination, the client complains to the nurse that she has pain in her left calf. The nurse should

   *A. examine both legs.
   B. apply pressure to the left calf area.
   C. ask the client if she has varicosities.
   D. have the client move the leg in an upward motion.

   Reference: p. 478

   Descriptors: 1. 26   2. 03   3. Application
                4. 5 = Implementation 5. Easy

8. During a health assessment, the client indicates to the nurse that she has a small mass on her wrist. To assess whether or not the mass is fluid-filled, the nurse palpates with the

   A. palm of the hand.
   B. fingernails of one hand.
   *C. fingers and finger pads.
   D. dorsal surface of the hand.

   Reference: p. 479

   Descriptors: 1. 26   2. 03   3. Application
                4. 2 = Assessment   5. Easy

9. While performing a health assessment of an adult client, the nurse exercises utmost caution when using

   *A. deep palpation.
   B. intermittant palpation.
   C. light palpation.
   D. surface palpation.

   Reference: p. 479

   Descriptors: 1. 26   2. 03   3. Application
                4. 5 = Implementation 5. Moderate

10. The nurse is planning to percuss a client's stomach to assess for tympany. ~~The nurse should~~ *What is the technique utilized to percuss?*
    A. place the dominant hand over the area and strike with forefinger.
    *B. use the middle finger of the dominant hand as the striking force.
    C. use both hands to determine vibration in the stomach area.
    D. place the client's dominant hand over the stomach area.

    Reference: p. 480

    Descriptors: 1. 26   2. 03   3. Application
                 4. 5 = Implementation 5. Moderate

11. The nurse determines that an adult client has a very loud, low-pitched sound with a booming quality over the left lung. The nurse documents this as

    A. tympany.
    B. resonance.
    *C. hyperresonance.
    D. hollowness.

    Reference: p. 480

    Descriptors: 1. 26   2. 08   3. Application
                 4. 3 = Analysis/Diag.   5. Moderate

12. The nurse performed a health assessment on a 79-year-old client. The nurse documents which of the following findings as abnormal for a client of this age?

    A. Decreased skin turgor
    B. Dry mucous membrane
    C. Tympany over the abdomen.
    *D. Jaundiced skin.

    Reference: p. 482

    Descriptors: 1. 26   2. 08   3. Application
                 4. 3 = Analysis   5. Moderate

13. The nurse assesses a dark-skinned client for cyanosis by observing the color of the

   *A. mucous membrane of the mouth.
   B. sclera of the eye.
   C. skin around the head and neck.
   D. toenails of the feet.

   Reference: p. 483

   Descriptors: 1. 26   2. 03   3. Application
                4. 2 = Assessment   5. Moderate

14. The nurse is perfoming a health assessment on a 10-year-old child. The nurse observes a purplish discoloration on the child's left knee. The nurse should document this as

   A. petechiae.
   B. lesions.
   C. desquamation.
   *D. ecchymosis.

   Reference: p. 483

   Descriptors: 1. 26   2. 08   3. Application
                4. 2 = Assessment   5. Easy

15. An adult client tells the nurse during a health assessment that he has had vitiligo for several years. The nurse anticipates that the client will have

   A. dark mucous membranes.
   *B. white patchy areas on the skin.
   C. erythema of the face.
   D. pallor in the conjunctivae.

   Reference: p. 483

   Descriptors: 1. 26   2. 08   3. Application
                4. 3 = Analysis/Diag.   5. Moderate

16. The nurse conducts a health assessment on an 18-year-old male and observes fissures in both feet. The nurse should ask the client if he has ever been treated for

   *A. athlete's foot.
   B. impetigo.
   C. allergies.
   D. wheals.

   Reference: p. 484

   Descriptors: 1. 26   2. 08   3. Application
                4. 3 = Analysis/Diag.   5. Moderate

17. While performing a physical assessment of a 76-year-old client, the nurse notes that the angle between the skin and the nail bed is flat and at 180°, with the skin tissue feeling springy and floating. The nurse documents this as

   A. spoon nails.
   B. onycholysis.
   *C. early clubbing.
   D. late clubbing.

   Reference: p. 485

   Descriptors: 1. 26   2. 08   3. Application
                4. 3 = Analysis/Diag.   5. Moderate

18. While inspecting the eyes of a hospitalized client, the nurse observes that the client has unequal pupils. The nurse determines that this is symptomatic of

   A. glaucoma.
   B. cataracts.
   C. blindness.
   *D. central nervous system injury.

   Reference: p. 487

   Descriptors: 1. 26   2. 08   3. Application
                4. 3 = Analysis/Diag.   5. Easy

19. To assess an adult client's consensual reflex, the nurse should

   *A. shine a penlight on one pupil and then the other.
   B. hold a pencil about 4 inches from the client's nose.
   C. move one finger towards the client's nose.
   D. use an ophthalmoscope to find the optic nerve.

   Reference: p. 487

   Descriptors: 1. 26   2. 05   3. Application
                4. 2 = Assessment   5. Moderate

20. The nurse is planning to assess a 30-month-old client who has had frequent ear infections. The nurse plans to

   A. use the smallest otoscope speculum that will fit the client's ear.
   B. instruct the mother to hold the client's head downward.
   C. straighten the ear canal by gently pulling the pinna up and back.
   *D. straighten the ear canal by gently pulling the pinna down and back.

   Reference: p. 490

   Descriptors: 1. 26   2. 07   3. Application
                4. 4 = Planning   5. Moderate

21. The nurse explains the purpose of Weber's test to an adult client. The nurse determines that the client has understood the instructions when the client says,

   *A. "This test is used to test bone conduction."
   B. "This test is used to test air conduction."
   C. "You will place the tuning fork close to my ear."
   D. "You will place the tuning fork at the back of my head."

   Reference: p. 491

   Descriptors: 1. 26   2. 04   3. Application
                4. 6 = Evaluation   5. Moderate

22. The nurse has completed a physical examination of an adult client's head and neck. Which of the following would be considered an abnormal finding?

   A. Small pink symmetrical tonsils.
   B. Palpable thyroid gland.
   *C. Neck vein distention.
   D. Nonpalpable lymph nodes.

   Reference: p. 493

   Descriptors: 1. 26   2. 08   3. Factual
              4. 3 = Analysis   5. Easy

23. While auscultating lung sounds, the nurse hears a grating sound. The nurse documents this finding as

   *A. pleural friction rub.
   B. gurgles.
   C. crackles.
   D. bronchiole rales.

   Reference: p. 497

   Descriptors: 1. 26   2. 08   3. Factual
              4. 3 = Analysis/Diag.   5. Moderate

24. In order to auscultate cardiac sounds and hear the S1 sound most clearly, the nurse plans to place the stethoscope at the area known as

   A. aortic.
   B. pulmonic.
   C. ventricular.
   *D. apical.

   Reference: p. 501

   Descriptors: 1. 26   2. 03   3. Factual
              4. 4 = Planning   5. Moderate

25. The nurse is preparing to perform a vaginal examination and obtain specimens of an adult client. After explaining the procedure to the client the nurse should *first*

   A. apply a water-soluble lubricant.
   *B. warm the speculum with warm water.
   C. shave the pubic hair.
   D. observe for lesions on the cervical os.

   Reference: p. 507

   Descriptors: 1. 26   2. 07   3. Application
              4. 5 = Implementation 5. Moderate

26. The nurse plans to assess a client's vagus nerve by asking the client to

   A. shrug the shoulders against the nurse's resistance.
   B. protrude the tongue forward.
   C. raise the eyebrows.
   *D. swallow and speak.

   Reference: p. 513

   Descriptors: 1. 26   2. 07   3. Factual
              4. 5 = Implementation 5. Moderate

27. During a health assessment, the nurse asks the client to open and clench her jaws in order to assess the

   A. abducens nerve.
   B. facial nerve.
   *C. trigeminal nerve.
   D. accessory nerve.

   Reference: p. 513

   Descriptors: 1. 26   2. 07   3. Factual
              4. 2 = Assessment   5. Moderate

28. The nurse is planning to assess a 79-year-old client with severe rheumatoid arthritis. The client is coherent and very talkative. A priority nursing diagnosis for this client is

   A. decisional conflict related to test outcomes.
   *B. high risk for injury related to limited mobility.
   C. anxiety related to perception of diagnostic treatments.
   D. knowledge deficit related to unfamiliarity of outcomes.

   Reference: p. 518

   Descriptors: 1. 26   2. 09   3. Application
              4. 3 = Analysis/Diag.   5. Moderate

29. A client is seen in the outpatient clinic and requests a test for HIV. Before collecting a sample for the test, the nurse should

   A. don sterile gloves.
   B. ask why the test is requested.
   C. provide a pamphlet about the test.
   *D. ask the client to sign an informed consent.

   Reference: p. 519

   Descriptors: 1. 26   2. 09   3. Application
              4. 5 = Implementation 5. Moderate

30. The nurse has instructed an adult client about nuclear scanning for a possible brain tumor. The nurse determines that the client understands the instructions when the client says

   A. "I will be without food or fluids for 8 hours after the test."
   B. "This test is similar to having a chest x-ray."
   C. "High frequency sounds are used in this test."
   *D. "I will receive a radionuclide for this test."

   Reference: p. 521

   Descriptors: 1. 26   2. 09   3. Application
              4. 6 = Evaluation   5. Moderate

CHAPTER 27
Safety

1. The nurse is caring for a pregnant client in the clinic when the client tells the nurse that she is trying to stop smoking. The nurse instructs the client that smoking while pregnant can lead to

   A. severe congenital anomalies.
   B. increased bleeding after delivery.
   C. decreased weight gain during pregnancy.
   *D. low birth weight in the newborn.

   Reference: p. 526

   Descriptors: 1. 27   2. 02   3. Application
   4. 5 = Implementation 5. Moderate

2. The nurse is planning to instruct a group of high school students on the topic of safety. Which of the following would be important to include in the teaching plan?

   *A. Many motor vehicle accident fatalities are alcohol-related.
   B. Domestic violence is common in this age group.
   C. Sports injuries are the primary cause of fatalities.
   D. Falls contribute to a majority of injuries in this age group.

   Reference: p. 526

   Descriptors: 1. 27   2. 02   3. Application
   4. 4 = Planning   5. Moderate

3. The nurse has presented a class to a group of adults age 65 or older on the topic of safety. The nurse determines that one of the members of the group needs further instructions when he says,

   A. "Domestic violence is frequently not reported."
   B. "Slowing reflexes can contribute to auto accidents."
   C. "More women than men have injuries due to falls."
   *D. "The typical victim of abuse is a male over the age of 70 years."

   Reference: p. 526

   Descriptors: 1. 27   2. 02   3. Application
   4. 6 = Evaluation   5. Moderate

4. A nurse working in an operating room has just learned that she is pregnant. The nurse should

   *A. consider a temporary transfer to another area of the health care facility.
   B. use caution when administering intravenous fluids.
   C. discontinue seat belt use until after delivery.
   D. take frequent rest breaks after lengthy operations.

   Reference: p. 527

   Descriptors: 1. 27   2. 02   3. Application
   4. 1 = No Process   5. Moderate

5. The nurse makes a home visit to an 86-year-old client with limited financial resources. While discussing fire safety with the client, the nurse should first assess

   A. how the client plans to escape a fire.
   *B. how the client heats the house.
   C. the frequency of checking the smoke detector.
   D. if the client knows the telephone number for emergencies.

   Reference: p. 530

   Descriptors: 1. 27   2. 02   3. Application
   4. 2 = Assessment   5. Moderate

6. An 85-year-old female client has returned home following hip replacement surgery. She uses a walker for ambulation. A priority nursing diagnosis is

   *A. risk of falling related to altered gait and posture.
   B. anxiety related to limited ambulation.
   C. potential for injury related to visual sensory deficit.
   D. situational conflict related to prior hospitalization.

   Reference: p. 530

   Descriptors: 1. 27   2. 07   3. Application
   4. 3 = Analysis/Diag.   5. Moderate

7. The nurse is planning a class related to safety issues for children for a group of new mothers. Which of the following would be important to include in the teaching plan?

   A. Small pillows may be used for infants in their cribs.
   B. Young children can play with plastic bags if they are carefully supervised.
   C. Carbon monoxide poisoning is common among young children.
   *D. Drowning is a common cause of mortality among young children.

   Reference: p. 530

   Descriptors: 1. 27   2. 02   3. Application
   4. 4 = Planning   5. Moderate

8. A confused 78-year-old client who has fallen three times in the past month is admitted to the hospital with a possible fractured hip. The priority nursing diagnosis for this client is

   A. impaired home maintenance management related to falls.
   B. anxiety related to possible outcomes and hospitalization.
   C. potential for suffocation related to confusion.
   *D. risk for trauma related to history of falls and confusion.

   Reference: p. 534

   Descriptors: 1. 27   2. 07   3. Application
   4. 3 = Analysis/Diag.   5. Moderate

9. The nurse has instructed a new mother about infant car seats. The nurse determines that the client understood the instructions when she says,

   *A. "I should use a rear-facing car seat placed in the back seat of the car."
    B. "A rear-facing car seat can be used in the front seat if I have a car with airbags."
    C. "There are some states in the U.S. that do not require that infant car seats be used."
    D. "If my child is over 20 pounds, the child can use a seat belt."

Reference: p. 538

Descriptors: 1. 27   2. 03   3. Application
               4. 6 = Evaluation   5. Moderate

10. The nurse is assessing a 4-year-old child while the mother is nearby. The nurse should explain to the mother that a major safety threat for preschoolers is

    A. auto injuries.
    B. ingestion of small parts of toys.
   *C. ingestion of poisons.
    D. flammable toys.

Reference: p. 538

Descriptors: 1. 27   2. 02   3. Application
               4. 5 = Implementation 5. Moderate

11. The nurse is caring for an 80-year-old apparently healthy client who has recently moved in with his 50-year-old son. The nurse plans to discuss safety issues with the son. Which of the following should be included in the nurse's teaching plan?

    A. Throw rugs should have non-skid backing.
    B. All medications should be locked up.
    C. A cane would be useful to prevent falls.
   *D. A night light should be on in the bathroom.

Reference: p. 540

Descriptors: 1. 27   2. 05   3. Application
               4. 4 = Planning   5. Moderate

12. The nurse has instructed a group of certified nursing assistants about the use of restraints within the health care facility. The nurse determines that one of the assistants needs *further* instructions when she says,

   *A. "Using restraints on confused clients usually leads to fewer falls."
    B. "In some situations, restraints may be the only solution."
    C. "There is danger of suffocation when restraints are used."
    D. "Pressure ulcers and fractures have been associated with use of restraints."

Reference: p. 541

Descriptors: 1. 27   2. 03   3. Application
               4. 6 = Evaluation   5. Moderate

13. The nurse removes the vest restraint of an 84-year-old client. While the client is free of the restraint, the nurse plans to

    A. keep the restraint tied to the bedrails.
    B. feed the client a snack or fruit juice.
    C. discuss why the restraint is necessary.
   *D. encourage the client to exercise.

Reference: p. 543

Descriptors: 1. 27   2. 05   3. Application
               4. 4 = Planning   5. Easy

14. The nurse discovers a small fire in a bathroom in a client's hospital room. After evacuating the clients from the room, the nurse should

    A. pour water on the fire quickly.
   *B. activate the hospital's fire code system.
    C. call the fire department.
    D. place wet sheets under the closed door.

Reference: p. 544

Descriptors: 1. 27   2. 08   3. Application
               4. 5 = Implementation 5. Easy

15. The nurse has instructed a group of elementary students about fire safety in the home. The nurse determines that one of the students needs *further* instructions when the student says,

   *A. "If my clothes are on fire, I should run outside."
    B. "Evacuate the house as soon as smoke is detected."
    C. "There should be a working smoke detector on every level."
    D. "I should cover my mouth with a wet cloth while exiting the house."

Reference: p. 544

Descriptors: 1. 27   2. 08   3. Application
               4. 6 = Evaluation   5. Easy

16. The nurse is working in a rehabilitation center where several of the clients are restrained. The nurse suggests to the employees that an alternative to a vest restraint is

    A. maintaining the client's bed in a high position.
    B. providing cool beverages close to the client's bed.
    C. reducing pain medication administration.
   *D. using pillows wedged against the side of the chair.

Reference: p. 544

Descriptors: 1. 27   2. 06   3. Application
               4. 5 = Implementation 5. Moderate

17. The nurse is counseling a young mother whose 3-year-old child has just been treated for an overdose of children's aspirin. The nurse determines that the mother needs *further* instructions when she says,

   *A. "I should lock up all medicines except the vitamins."
   B. "Toxic plants such as holly berry can be dangerous."
   C. "I should keep all laundry products out of reach."
   D. "After a medication is expired, I should dispose of it down the sink."

   Reference: pp. 547, 549

   Descriptors: 1. 27   2. 09   3. Application
                4. 6 = Evaluation   5. Moderate

18. The nurse is caring for a 70-year-old client who is taking numerous daily medications for arthritis, hypertension, and a urinary tract infection. The nurse should suggest that the client

   A. take the medicine for arthritis first to relieve pain.
   B. take all of the daily medications at the same time.
   C. stop taking a prescription drug if there are side effects.
   *D. use a medication calendar or diary to keep track of the medications.

   Reference: p. 549

   Descriptors: 1. 27   2. 03   3. Application
                4. 5 = Implementation 5. Moderate

19. The nurse is completing an incident report after a hospitalized client received an incorrect medication. The nurse plans to

   A. document who administered the incorrect medication.
   *B. provide details about the client's response after the incident.
   C. send the incident report to the medical records department after it is completed.
   D. ask the physician to document the client's condition in the medical record after the incident.

   Reference: p. 551

   Descriptors: 1. 27   2. 03   3. Application
                4. 4 = Planning   5. Moderate

20. While assessing a client with an electronic monitoring device, the nurse detects a slight tingling sensation from the equipment. The nurse should

   *A. report the faulty equipment to the appropriate department.
   B. check to see if the equipment has a three-prong plug.
   C. determine whether the electrodes are correctly applied.
   D. place the equipment in the utility room.

   Reference: p. 550

   Descriptors: 1. 27   2. 03   3. Application
                4. 5 = Implementation 5. Moderate

CHAPTER 28
Asepsis

1. The nurse is caring for a postoperative client with a temperature of 103.6°F. After collecting a blood specimen for a culture, which of the following will most likely be ordered by the client's physician?

   A. Gram-positive
   B. Gram-negative
   C. Antifungal
   *D. Broad-spectrum

   Reference: p. 556

   Descriptors: 1. 28   2. 01   3. Application
                4. 1 = No Process   5. Moderate

2. A client is seen in the emergency room following an outdoor picnic and is diagnosed with food poisoning. The nurse should explain to the client that this type of infection is transmitted in which of the following ways?

   *A. Vehicle
   B. Vector
   C. Airborne
   D. Direct contact

   Reference: p. 557

   Descriptors: 1. 28   2. 02   3. Factual
                4. 5 = Implementation 5. Moderate

3. The nurse has instructed a group of health care workers about prevention of the virus that transmits hepatitis B. The nurse determines that one of the workers needs *further* instructions when she says that the virus is transmitted by

   A. blood.
   B. feces.
   C. bodily fluids.
   *D. sputum.

   Reference: p. 558

   Descriptors: 1. 28   2. 02   3. Application
                4. 6 = Evaluation   5. Moderate

4. A 74-year-old female client is diagnosed with chronic urinary tract infections. The nurse plans to instruct the client that one of the reasons for increased urinary tract infections in older adults is that

A. there is less intact skin.
*B. the bladder is not completely emptied.
C. the pH of the urethra is increased.
D. there is an increased inflammatory response.

Reference: p. 559

Descriptors: 1. 28   2. 05   3. Application
            4. 4 = Planning   5. Moderate

5. A 75-year-old client is hospitalized with pneumonia and a urinary tract infection. The client has an indwelling urinary catheter and appears malnourished. The nurse caring for the client determines that the client's priority nursing diagnosis is

A. risk for chronic infections due to advanced age.
*B. risk for infection related to malnutrition.
C. potential for immobility related to urinary catheter.
D. social isolation related to presence of disease.

Reference: p. 560

Descriptors: 1. 28   2. 08   3. Interpretive
            4. 3 = Analysis/Diag.   5. Moderate

6. A 45-year-old client is preparing for discharge from the hospital when the client develops a temperature of 102.8°F. The nurse determines that the client is experiencing an infection termed

*A. nosocomial.
B. extracorporeal.
C. incidental.
D. resistant.

Reference: p. 561

Descriptors: 1. 28   2. 01   3. Application
            4. 3 = Analysis   5. Moderate

7. A 60-year-old client has had an indwelling urinary catheter for two days following surgery. Before removing the catheter, the nurse sends a urine sample for analysis, culture, and sensitivity to determine if the client has developed an infection termed

A. endogenous.
B. viral.
C. microbial.
*D. iatrogenic.

Reference: p. 561

Descriptors: 1. 28   2. 01   3. Factual
            4. 5 = Implementation   5. Moderate

8. The nurse has conducted a class for health care workers on the topic of infection control. The nurse determines that one of the workers needs *further* instructions when he says,

A. "Most hospital-acquired infections are due to bacteria."
B. "Indwelling catheters have been implicated in a large percentage of infections."
*C. "Hospital-acquired infections are relatively easy to treat with antibiotics."
D "Frequent handwashing is the best method of preventing hospital-acquired infections."

Reference: p. 561

Descriptors: 1. 28   2. 03   3. Application
            4. 6 = Evaluation   5. Moderate

9. A hospitalized client has developed a severe enterococcal infection following abdominal surgery. The nurse anticipates that the physician will order the drug

A. methicillin.
B. penicillin.
C. streptomycin.
*D. vancomycin.

Reference: p. 561

Descriptors: 1. 28   2. 06   3. Application
            4. 1 = No Process   5. Moderate

10. The nurse has instructed a group of newly employed nursing assistants about medical asepsis. The nurse assesses the workers during morning care to determine if medical asepsis techniques are broken by the employee who

A. keeps soiled linens away from her clothing.
*B. places soiled linens on the floor near the client.
C. uses a dampened cloth to dust the bedside table.
D. cleans the least soiled area near the client first.

Reference: p. 562

Descriptors: 1. 28   2. 03   3. Application
            4. 1 = No Process   5. Moderate

11. Before changing a clean dressing of a home care client, the nurse should *first*

*A. wash the hands with an antibacterial soap.
B. remove any nail polish on the fingernails.
C. put on two pairs of clean gloves.
D. remove any wedding rings or other jewelry.

Reference: p. 563

Descriptors: 1. 28   2. 07   3. Application
            4. 5 = Implementation 5. Easy

12. The nurse is working in a gynecologic clinic. Before sending contaminated specula to the central supply area the nurse plans to be certain that the items are

A. washed first in hot soapy water.
B. sent in a basin of warm soapy water.
C. placed in a bag designated for blood and bodily fluids.
*D. rinsed first in cold running water.

Reference: p. 566

Descriptors: 1. 28   2. 03   3. Application
           4. 4 = Planning   5. Moderate

13. The nurse is caring for a 78-year-old client at home with a postoperative abdominal dressing. The nurse assesses the client and determines that the technique used for this dressing change should be

A. clean.
B. antiseptic.
*C. sterile.
D. medically aseptic.

Reference: p. 566

Descriptors: 1. 28   2. 10   3. Application
           4. 2 = Assessment   5. Easy

14. The nurse is caring for a client at home diagnosed with HIV infection. The nurse should instruct the client that an effective disinfectant for home use is

A. alcohol.
*B. household bleach.
C. boiling water.
D. providine.

Reference: p. 567

Descriptors: 1. 28   2. 03   3. Application
           4. 5 = Implementation 5. Moderate

15. The nurse assesses a sterile field and determines that it has been contaminated when the nurse observes

A. the outer 1 inch of the sterile towel over the side of the table.
B. sterile objects held above the waist of the practitioner.
C. sterile packages opened so that the first edge is away from the practitioner.
*D. wetness on the sterile cloth on top of a non-sterile table.

Reference: p. 565

Descriptors: 1. 28   2. 10   3. Application
           4. 6 = Evaluation   5. Moderate

16. The nurse is preparing to perform a normal saline wet-to-dry dressing change on a home care client. The nurse notes that the capped, partially used bottle at the client's bedside was opened 4 hours earlier. The nurse should

*A. discard a small amount of the solution into the sink prior to using the solution.
B. ask the client if the bottle was really opened only 4 hours ago.
C. throw away the old bottle and open a new one before the dressing change.
D. clean the inside of the cap with sterile water before putting the cap on a sterile area.

Reference: p. 568

Descriptors: 1. 28   2. 10   3. Application
           4. 5 = Implementation 5. Moderate

17. An adult client has been instructed on the use of sterile technique to change his dressing. During a return demonstration, the nurse determines that the client has understood the instructions when the client

A. puts on sterile gloves before beginning the procedure.
B. places the solution container at the back of the sterile field.
C. opens the dressing package and drops it from a height of 15 inches.
*D. opens the sterile packages before donning the sterile gloves.

Reference: p. 570

Descriptors: 1. 28   2. 10   3. Application
           4. 6 = Evaluation   5. Moderate

18. The nurse is planning to remove sterile gloves following a wet-to-dry dressing change. The nurse plans to

*A. use the dominant hand to grasp the other glove on the outside of the cuff.
B. use the non-dominant hand to grasp the other glove at the fingertips.
C. grasp the glove on the non-dominant hand on the inside of the cuff.
D. wash both hands with an antimicrobial solution before removal.

Reference: p. 575

Descriptors: 1. 28   2. 10   3. Application
           4. 4 = Planning   5. Moderate

19. The nurse has instructed a group of new employees about universal precautions. The nurse determines that one of the employees needs *further* instructions when he says that universal precautions are necessary when handling items that are soiled with

   *A. sweat.
   B. amnionic fluid.
   C. cerebrospinal fluid.
   D. vaginal secretions.

   Reference: p. 576

   Descriptors:　1. 28　　2. 09　　3. Application
   　　　　　　　4. 6 = Evaluation　5. Moderate

20. The nurse is notified that a client with hepatitis A will soon be admitted to the hospital unit. The nurse determines that this client will require

   A. respiratory isolation.
   *B. enteric precautions.
   C. contact precautions.
   D. strict isolation.

   Reference: p. 577

   Descriptors:　1. 28　　2. 09　　3. Application
   　　　　　　　4. 4 = Planning　5. Moderate

21. The nurse provides directions to a nursing assistant who will be changing soiled bed linens of a client with pneumonia. The nurse should instruct the nursing assistant to wear

   *A. sterile gloves.
   B. a mask.
   C. a clean gown.
   D. clean gloves.

   Reference: p. 577

   Descriptors:　1. 28　　2. 09　　3. Application
   　　　　　　　4. 5 = Implementation 5. Moderate

22. The nurse is caring for several adult clients on a hospital unit. For which one of the following clients would the nurse plan to practice strict isolation? A client diagnosed with

   *A. smallpox.
   B. pneumonia.
   C. hepatitis B.
   D. malaria.

   Reference: p. 577

   Descriptors:　1. 28　　2. 09　　3. Application
   　　　　　　　4. 4 = Planning　5. Moderate

23. A client has been admitted to the hospital and is diagnosed with vancomycin-resistant enterococci (VRE). The nurse plans to instruct the client that

   A. the client will most likely have no visitors allowed.
   B. all health care workers will wear masks before entering the room.
   C. sterile gloves will be used when providing care.
   *D. frequently used equipment will be kept in the room.

   Reference: p. 579

   Descriptors:　1. 28　　2. 10　　3. Application
   　　　　　　　4. 4 = Planning　5. Moderate

24. The nurse is supervising a nursing student who is preparing to provide care for a client with active tuberculosis. Before assisting the student in providing care to this client, the nurse assesses the student's awareness of the necessity for wearing

   *A. masks.
   B. sterile gloves.
   C. clean gowns.
   D. clean gloves.

   Reference: p. 580

   Descriptors:　1. 28　　2. 09　　3. Application
   　　　　　　　4. 2 = Assessment　5. Moderate

25. An infection control nurse becomes concerned when she observes

   A. double bagging of soiled linens.
   B. securely tied plastic trash bags.
   *C. a leaking urine specimen placed in a basket.
   D. clean gloves being worn by laundry personnel.

   Reference: p. 581

   Descriptors:　1. 28　　2. 09　　3. Application
   　　　　　　　4. 1 = No Process　5. Moderate

26. While caring for a client who has intermittent diarrhea, the nurse plans to take precautions to prevent contamination from

   *A. *Escherichia coli.*
   B. *Clostridium difficile.*
   C. *Staphylococcus aureus.*
   D. *Neisseria menigitidis.*

   Reference: p. 582

   Descriptors:　1. 28　　2. 09　　3. Factual
   　　　　　　　4. 4 = Planning　5. Moderate

27. The nurse has demonstrated how to don sterile gloves to a group of nursing students. The nurse should instruct the students that

A. vinyl glove punctures reseal automatically.
B. latex gloves are used primarily with minor procedures.
C. vinyl gloves are less costly and easier to put on.
*D. latex gloves can result in allergic reactions.

Reference: p. 585

Descriptors: 1. 28   2. 10   3. Application
4. 5 = Implementation 5. Moderate

28. The nurse is planning to assist another nurse to perform tracheostomy suctioning. Before beginning the procedure, the nurse plans to

A. double-bag all used equipment.
B. obtain a particulate respirator mask.
*C. wear protective eyewear with sideshields.
D. put on a sterile gown.

Reference: pp. 586–587

Descriptors: 1. 28   2. 10   3. Application
4. 4 = Planning   5. Moderate

29. A client has been placed in isolation because he is diagnosed with a contagious illness. The nurse should instruct the client that

A. linens from the client's bed will be double-bagged.
*B. meals will be served on washable dishes.
C. extensive isolation rarely causes psychological problems.
D. paper trays and plastic utensils prevent disease transmission.

Reference: p. 587

Descriptors: 1. 28   2. 10   3. Application
4. 5 = Implementation 5. Moderate

30. The nurse receives a needlestick following administration of an injection to a client. The nurse should *first*

*A. wash the exposed area with soap and warm water.
B. report the incident to the appropriate person.
C. receive a blood test to determine his/her HIV status.
D. ask the client to consent to an HIV blood test.

Reference: p. 589

Descriptors: 1. 28   2. 09   3. Application
4. 5 = Implementation 5. Moderate

CHAPTER 29
Medications

1. The law which was enacted in 1970 to regulate the distribution of narcotics and other drugs of abuse is known as the

A. Comprehensive Food, Drug, and Cosmetic Act.
B. Federal Narcotic and Abuse Act.
C. Pure Food and Drug Act.
*D. Controlled Substances Act.

Reference: p. 594

Descriptors: 1. 29   2. 02   3. Factual
4. 1 = No Process   5. Easy

2. When different manufacturers produce the same drug, the drug is usually sold by its

A. generic name.
*B. brand name.
C. chemical name.
D. official name.

Reference: p. 595

Descriptors: 1. 29   2. 01   3. Factual
4. 1 = No Process   5. Easy

3. An adult client has an elixir medication ordered. The nurse should explain to the client that elixir medications

A. allow for slow release over a period of time.
B. should be shaken briefly before injection.
*C. have a clear liquid with water, alcohol, and flavoring.
D. should be dissolved slowly in the mouth for 10 minutes.

Reference: p. 596

Descriptors: 1. 29   2. 01   3. Application
4. 5 = Implementation 5. Moderate

4. The nurse has explained aqueous solution medications to the client in the home care setting. The nurse determines that the client understands the instructions when the client says,

*A. "My medication has been dissolved in water."
B. "This medication is dissolved in water and sugar."
C. "Absorption through the skin is how the medication works."
D. "I should shake the container well before taking this medication."

Reference: p. 596

Descriptors: 1. 29   2. 03   3. Application
4. 6 = Evaluation   5. Moderate

5. The nurse is caring for a client who is approximately 4 months pregnant. The nurse plans to explain to the client that drugs taken while pregnant

   A. will cause harmful effects on the fetus.
   B. should be in a water-soluble form.
   C. can affect the rate of the client's metabolism.
   *D. have the potential for harmful effects on the fetus.

   Reference: pp. 597, 598

   Descriptors: 1. 29   2. 05   3. Application
            4. 4 = Planning   5. Moderate

6. The primary site for drug metabolism is the

   *A. liver.
   B. brain.
   C. kidneys.
   D. intestines.

   Reference: p. 597

   Descriptors: 1. 29   2. 01   3. Factual
            4. 1 = No Process   5. Easy

7. The nurse is caring for a 68-year-old client in the home. The client is taking several prescription drugs on a daily basis. While caring for the client, the nurse should assess the client's

   A. ability to metabolize the drugs.
   B. liver functions studies.
   *C. over the counter drug use.
   D. capillary blood flow.

   Reference: p. 598

   Descriptors: 1. 29   2. 05   3. Application
            4. 2 = Assessment   5. Moderate

8. A 10-year-old child weighing 113 pounds has an order for Demerol 75 mg IM q. 3–4 h following abdominal surgery. The nurse determines that

   *A. this dosage is appropriate for this child's weight.
   B. this dosage of medication is not recommended for a 10-year-old child.
   C. lower pain tolerances in children of this age require strong pain medications.
   D. the absorption rate of Demerol requires increased dosage following surgery.

   Reference: p. 598

   Descriptors: 1. 29   2. 05   3. Application
            4. 3 = Analysis/Diag.   5. Moderate

9. A 72-year-old client has been taking an oral beta blocker medication for hypertension for 7 days. The nurse should assess the client for

   A. increased weight gain.
   B. stomach irritation.
   C. diarrhea or runny stools.
   *D. dizziness or lightheadedness.

   Reference: p. 598

   Descriptors: 1. 29   2. 05   3. Application
            4. 2 = Assessment   5. Moderate

10. The nurse is caring for an Asian-American client weighing 100 pounds who has been given a prescription for an antihypertensive medication. The nurse should instruct the client that

    *A. herbal remedies may interfere with the drug's action.
    B. small body weight and size may result in unexpected side effects.
    C. enzyme deficiencies common in Asian-American clients may cause drug reactions.
    D. the medication should be decreased when the client's blood pressure is normal.

    Reference: p. 599

    Descriptors: 1. 29   2. 05   3. Application
             4. 5 = Implementation 5. Moderate

11. An hour after administration of oral penicillin, an adult client complains to the nurse that he has a rash over his arms and abdomen. The nurse determines that the client is most likely experiencing a reaction to the drug termed

    A. anaphylaxis.
    B. idiosyncratic.
    C. antagonistic.
    *D. allergy.

    Reference: p. 600

    Descriptors: 1. 29   2. 05   3. Interpretive
             4. 3 = Analysis/Diag.   5. Easy

12. A few minutes after receiving an injection of penicillin, a client complains of chest pain and dyspnea. The nurse notifies the physician as this client is most likely experiencing a reaction termed

    A. idiosyncratic.
    B. overdose.
    *C. anaphylaxis
    D. synergistic.

    Reference: p. 600

    Descriptors: 1. 29   2. 05   3. Interpretive
             4. 3 = Analysis/Diag.   5. Moderate

13. A 69-year-old client has been taking 2 mg of Valium twice daily for several months. In the past few days, the client has become very agitated and restless. The nurse determines that the client is experiencing a drug reaction termed

    *A. idiosyncratic.
    B. cumulative.
    C. tolerant.
    D. synergistic.

    Reference: p. 600

    Descriptors: 1. 29   2. 05   3. Interpretive
             4. 3 = Analysis/Diag.   5. Moderate

14. While caring for a 74-year-old client in the home, the nurse determines that the client has not been taking his prescribed antibiotics correctly. The client complains to the nurse that the drug costs "too much money, and makes me nauseated." A priority nursing diagnosis for this client is

   A. knowledge deficit related to medication regimen.
   B. altered health maintenance related to side effects of medications.
 *C. noncompliance with medication regimen related to costs.
   D. risk for aspiration related to age and side effects of drug.

Reference: p. 600

Descriptors: 1. 29   2. 08   3. Application
           4. 3 = Analysis/Diag. 5. Moderate

15. A 12-year-old client with epilepsy has been taking the drug Dilantin for several years to control seizures. The client is admitted to the hospital for surgery and the nurse discovers that the physician has not written any orders for Dilantin. The nurse plans to

 *A. contact the physician and request an order for Dilantin.
   B. allow the client to take her own Dilantin medication while hospitalized.
   C. tell the client's mother that she must take the client's Dilantin medication home with her.
   D. document in the nursing assessment record that the client has been taking Dilantin.

Reference: p. 601

Descriptors: 1. 29   2. 08   3. Application
           4. 4 = Planning   5. Moderate

16. The nurse is caring for a client who had surgery 6 hours ago. In checking the chart for a postoperative pain medication the nurse reviews the medication orders termed

   A. single.
   B. standing.
   C. stat.
 *D. PRN.

Reference: p. 602

Descriptors: 1. 29   2. 08   3. Application
           4. 5 = Implementation 5. Easy

17. The nurse is caring for a client who is receiving a narcotic medication for postoperative pain. In reviewing the doctor's order, the nurse should be certain that the order

   A. indicates what to do if a reaction occurs.
   B. offers several choices for pain medication.
   C. lists the possible allergic reactions.
 *D. has a valid date, time, and signature.

Reference: p. 603

Descriptors: 1. 29   2. 08   3. Application
           4. 1 = No Process   5. Moderate

18. An adult client is scheduled for surgery and the physician has ordered the preoperative medication. After the physician leaves the unit, the nurse discovers that the client has had an allergic reaction to this medication in the past. The nurse plans to

   A. administer the drug while observing the client for any reaction.
 *B. contact the physician and indicate that the client has had a previous reaction.
   C. ask the client how severe the reaction to the drug was in the past.
   D. withhold administration of the prescribed medication.

Reference: p. 605

Descriptors: 1. 29   2. 08   3. Application
           4. 4 = Planning   5. Moderate

19. While reading a physician's order, the nurse has difficulty reading the exact dosage prescribed because the handwriting is illegible. In this situation the nurse should

   A. ask the client what dosage was given in the past.
   B. ask another nurse to determine the correct dosage.
   C. tell the client that the medication will not be given.
 *D. contact the physician to determine the correct dosage.

Reference: p. 605

Descriptors: 1. 29   2. 08   3. Application
           4. 5 = Implementation 5. Easy

20. The physician has ordered the following medication for an adult client: "Isoflurophate 0.1% ophthalmic solution, instill ii gtt OD, bid." The nurse plans to administer this medication

 *A. in the right eye twice daily.
   B. in the left eye twice daily.
   C. in both eyes twice daily.
   D. in both eyes every other day.

Reference: p. 605

Descriptors: 1. 29   2. 08   3. Application
           4. 4 = Planning   5. Moderate

21. The physician has ordered that a client be given ASA 300 mg. tid pc. The nurse should administer the drug

   A. before meals.
 *B. after meals.
   C. twice daily.
   D. every three hours.

Reference: p. 605

Descriptors: 1. 29   2. 08   3. Application
           4. 5 = Implementation 5. Moderate

22. A client is prescribed Lanoxin 30 micrograms once daily. Available is Lanoxin 0.1 mg per mL. The nurse plans to administer

A. 0.003 mg.
*B. 0.03 mg.
C. 0.3 mg.
D. 3 mg.

Reference: p. 607

Descriptors: 1. 29   2. 07   3. Application
          4. 4 = Planning   5. Moderate

23. The physician orders Phenobarbital i grain. The medication is available in 30 milligram tablets. The nurse plans to administer

A. one tablet.
*B. two tablets.
C. three tablets.
D. four tablets.

Reference: p. 608

Descriptors: 1. 29   2. 07   3. Application
          4. 4 = Planning   5. Easy

24. The nurse is caring for a 7-year-old child on a pediatric unit. To calculate the appropriate medication dosage, the nurse uses the child's body surface area. The nurse should calculate the client's dosage by calculating the

*A. child's BSA divided by an adult's BSA times adult dose equals child's dose.
B. usual adult dose times the weight of the child divided by 150 equals child's dose.
C. adult's BSA divided by the child's BSA times adult dose equals child's dose.
D. child's BSA times the adult BSA divided by the adult dose equals child's dose.

Reference: p. 608

Descriptors: 1. 29   2. 07   3. Application
          4. 5 = Implementation 5. Moderate

25. While preparing a medication for an adult client, the nurse should read the label of the medication container

A. one time.
B. two times.
*C. three times.
D. four times.

Reference: p. 608

Descriptors: 1. 29   2. 08   3. Application
          4. 5 = Implementation 5. Moderate

26. The nurse has prepared an oral antibiotic medication for an adult client when the charge nurse tells her that she is needed immediately in another room. The nurse should

A. quickly administer the medication before going to another room.
*B. place the prepared medication in a locked medicine cart or cabinet.
C. ask another nurse to administer the prepared medication.
D. tell the client that the nurse is needed in another room.

Reference: p. 609

Descriptors: 1. 29   2. 08   3. Application
          4. 5 = Implementation 5. Moderate

27. While obtaining a narcotic pain medication for a hospitalized client, the nurse discovers that the narcotic count is incorrect. The nurse should

A. determine the cause of the discrepancy at the end of the shift.
B. notify the nursing chief of the hospital immediately.
C. ask another nurse if there was a discrepancy earlier in the shift.
*D. report the discrepancy to the charge nurse immediately.

Reference: p. 609

Descriptors: 1. 29   2. 08   3. Application
          4. 5 = Implementation 5. Moderate

28. The nurse has been caring for an adult client for the past 5 days on a rehabilitation unit. Before administering a prescribed antibiotic, the nurse plans to

*A. check the client's identification bracelet.
B. ask the visitor to state the client's name.
C. ask the client if she has any allergies to drugs.
D. check the chart at the client's bed for accuracy.

Reference: pp. 609, 612

Descriptors: 1. 29   2. 08   3. Application
          4. 4 = Planning   5. Easy

29. A hospitalized adult client has several oral medications ordered at the same time. The nurse should plan to

A. determine if the client can receive all of the medications at once.
B. leave the medications at the bedside if the client is in the bathroom.
C. ask the physician if the client can be on a self-medication schedule.
*D. offer the client one medication at a time while remaining with the client.

Reference: p. 609

Descriptors: 1. 29   2. 08   3. Application
          4. 4 = Planning   5. Easy

30. The nurse has instructed an adult client about the enteric coated tablets ordered by the physician. The nurse determines that the client understands the instructions when the client says, "Enteric coated medications

    A. should be chewed before I swallow them."
    B. are irritating to the small intestines."
    *C. prevent stomach irritation."
    D. can be dissolved in a liquid before I swallow them."

    Reference: p. 610

    Descriptors: 1. 29   2. 09   3. Application
                 4. 6 = Evaluation   5. Moderate

31. The physician has ordered mineral oil for an adult client. To make this drug easier for the client to swallow, the nurse plans to

    *A. offer the client very cold mineral oil followed by a glass of orange juice.
    B. mix the mineral oil in grape juice before administering the drug.
    C. ask the client to take sips of warm water before the drug is administered.
    D. mix the mineral oil with lukewarm milk before administering the drug.

    Reference: p. 610

    Descriptors: 1. 29   2. 08   3. Application
                 4. 4 = Planning   5. Moderate

32. The nurse is caring for an 80-year-old client in the home. The client takes several medications on a daily basis. The nurse has instructed the client about medication safety and determines that the client needs *further* instructions when she says

    *A. "My medications are safe regardless of how old they are."
    B. "I can ask the pharmacist for non-child-proof caps."
    C. "Liquid medications that discolor my teeth can be taken with a straw."
    D. "I should check the name of the drug and not go by the color."

    Reference: p. 614

    Descriptors: 1. 29   2. 09   3. Application
                 4. 6 = Evaluation   5. Easy

33. The physician has ordered a medication for an adult client with a nasogastric tube. The nurse should first assess the client by

    A. flushing the tube with 15 mL of normal saline.
    B. asking a preference for cold or warm liquids.
    C. determining if the tube is connected to suction.
    *D. determining patency of the tube.

    Reference: p. 615

    Descriptors: 1. 29   2. 08   3. Application
                 4. 2 = Assessment   5. Moderate

34. An adult client has been prescribed nitroglycerin tablets for angina. The nurse has instructed the client about the correct route for the drug and determines that the client understands the instructions when he says the drug should be taken by which of the following routes?

    A. Oral
    B. Rectal
    C. Nasal
    *D. Sublingual

    Reference: p. 615

    Descriptors: 1. 29   2. 09   3. Application
                 4. 6 = Evaluation   5. Moderate

35. The nurse is planning to administer 2 mL of a viscous medication intramuscularly to an adult client who is 5 feet tall and weighs 155 pounds. The nurse plans to use a 3 mL syringe with a

    A. 5/8-inch 25-gauge needle.
    B. 1-inch 23-gauge needle.
    *C. 1 1/2-inch 21-gauge needle.
    D. 2-inch 14-gauge needle.

    Reference: p. 615

    Descriptors: 1. 29   2. 08   3. Application
                 4. 4 = Planning   5. Moderate

36. The nurse is caring for an adult client when the physician orders a medication that is supplied in a vial. Before drawing the medication into the syringe, the nurse should *first*

    A. break the thin neck of the container.
    B. discard 0.5 mL of the medication for sterility.
    C. remove the rubber stopper on the top of the vial.
    *D. inject an amount of air equal to the medication.

    Reference: p. 617

    Descriptors: 1. 29   2. 08   3. Application
                 4. 5 = Implementation   5. Moderate

37. The nurse has instructed a nursing student how to prepare an injection of two drugs from separate vials. The nurse determines that the student understands the instructions when the student says,

    *A. "I should change the needle before drawing the medication from the second vial."
    B. "I should inject air into the first vial, then draw up the medication."
    C. "Excess medication can be re-injected into the second vial."
    D. "If I have a vial and an ampule, I should draw up the medication from the ampule first."

    Reference: p. 617

    Descriptors: 1. 29   2. 08   3. Application
                 4. 6 = Evaluation   5. Moderate

38. When drawing up a medication from an ampule, the nurse should

 A. consider the rim of the ampule as sterile.
 *B. use a filter needle to withdraw the solution.
 C. wrap a paper towel around the neck of the ampule before breaking it.
 D. inject 0.5 mL of air into the ampule before withdrawing the medication.

 Reference: p. 618

 Descriptors: 1. 29   2. 08   3. Application
              4. 5 = Implementation 5. Moderate

39. A diabetic client has a physician's order for NPH insulin, 20 units, and Regular insulin, 10 units, bid. The nurse has instructed the client how to mix the two insulin medications in one syringe. The nurse determines that the client needs *further* instructions when the client

 A. withdraws the NPH insulin dose first.
 B. rotates the NPH vial before withdrawing the medication.
 C. touches the plunger of the syringe at only the knob.
 *D. withdraws the Regular insulin dose first.

 Reference: pp. 623–624

 Descriptors: 1. 29   2. 08   3. Application
              4. 6 = Evaluation   5. Moderate

40. The nurse is caring for a client who is scheduled for diagnostic testing which requires a lengthy absorption time of a particular medication. The nurse should explain to the client that the medication will be administered by the parenteral route termed

 A. intravenous.
 B. transdermal.
 *C. intradermal.
 D. subcutaneous.

 Reference: p. 624

 Descriptors: 1. 29   2. 08   3. Application
              4. 5 = Implementation 5. Moderate

41. The nurse has instructed a client how to administer heparin injections in the home setting. The nurse determines that the client needs *further* instructions when the nurse observes the client during the return demonstration

 *A. aspirate for blood before injecting the medication.
 B. rotate injection sites throughout the abdominal area.
 C. wash her hands following the injection.
 D. avoid massage of the site after the injection.

 Reference: p. 627

 Descriptors: 1. 29   2. 08   3. Application
              4. 6 = Evaluation   5. Moderate

42. The nurse is preparing to inject 2 mL of a viscous medication intramuscularly to an adult client. The nurse determines that the best site for the injection is the

 *A. ventrogluteal site.
 B. deltoid site.
 C. rectus femoris site.
 D. dorsogluteal site.

 Reference: pp. 631–632

 Descriptors: 1. 29   2. 08   3. Application
              4. 3 = Analysis/Diag.   5. Moderate

43. A nurse is preparing to administer a 1 mL vitamin K intramuscular injection to an infant weighing 7 pounds. The nurse determines that the best site for the injection is the

 A. dorsogluteal site.
 B. deltoid site.
 C. ventrogluteal site.
 *D. vastus lateralis site.

 Reference: p. 632

 Descriptors: 1. 29   2. 08   3. Application
              4. 3 = Analysis   5. Moderate

44. The nurse is preparing to administer iron dextran intramuscularly by the Z-track method. The nurse plans to

 A. put an air bubble at the tip of the syringe.
 *B. change the needle after withdrawing the medication.
 C. massage the site following the injection.
 D. quickly withdraw the needle following the injection.

 Reference: pp. 633, 636

 Descriptors: 1. 29   2. 08   3. Application
              4. 4 = Planning   5. Moderate

45. The physician prescribed an intravenous antibiotic for an adult client which is to be administered through a heparin lock. The nurse plans to

 A. connect the client to regular intravenous fluids after administration of the antibiotic.
 B. administer the medication as a bolus infusion.
 *C. flush the heparin lock with normal saline after the antibiotic is infused.
 D. administer intermittent infusions of heparin to maintain patency of the heparin lock.

 Reference: pp. 637, 641

 Descriptors: 1. 29   2. 08   3. Application
              4. 4 = Planning   5. Moderate

46. An adult client has a physician's order for an ointment to treat itching. To promote absorption of the drug the nurse should

A. apply an ice pack to the area after application.
*B. wash the area prior to application.
C. wear sterile gloves before application.
D. ask the client to remain in bed after the application.

Reference: p. 642

Descriptors: 1. 29   2. 08   3. Application
4. 5 = Implementation 5. Moderate

47. The nurse has instructed a home care client about the use of a transdermal nitroglycerin patch. During the return demonstration by the client, the nurse determines that the client understands the instructions when the nurse observes the client

*A. write the date and time on the patch.
B. place the new patch at the same location as the previous one.
C. leave the used patch on the bedside table.
D. place the patch over skin which is reddened and dry.

Reference: p. 649

Descriptors: 1. 29   2. 09   3. Application
4. 6 = Evaluation   5. Moderate

48. The nurse is preparing to administer eyedrops to an adult client. The nurse plans to

A. wear sterile gloves for the procedure.
B. ask the client to look down during the instillation.
C. cleanse the eyelids from the outer canthus to the inner canthus.
*D. administer the number of drops ordered into the conjunctival sac.

Reference: p. 650

Descriptors: 1. 29   2. 08   3. Application
4. 4 = Planning   5. Moderate

49. The nurse has instructed a family member of an adult client on the procedure for ear drop instillation for both ears. The nurse determines that the family member needs *further* instructions when the nurse observes the family member

A. clean the external ear with cotton balls moistened with saline.
B. turn the client to the unaffected side before instillation.
C. hold the dropper with its ear tip above the auditory canal.
*D. instill the drops into the second ear immediately after the first instillation.

Reference: p. 653

Descriptors: 1. 29   2. 09   3. Application
4. 6 = Evaluation   5. Moderate

50. The nurse has instructed an adult client how to instill nose drops that have been ordered by the physician. The nurse determines that the client understands the instructions when the client says,

*A. "I should blow my nose before instilling the drops."
B. "I should hold my head forward before instilling the drops."
C. "I should draw up enough medication for the first instillation and then draw up the second drops."
D. "I should place the dropper far back into the nose."

Reference: p. 655

Descriptors: 1. 29   2. 09   3. Application
4. 6 = Evaluation   5. Moderate

51. An adult client hospitalized for pneumonia refuses to take his oral antibiotics because the drugs make him feel nauseated. The nurse should

A. stay with the client until the medication is consumed.
B. tell the client that it is hospital policy that he cannot refuse the medication.
*C. report the client's refusal to the client's physician.
D. document the client's refusal on the client's Kardex.

Reference: p. 659

Descriptors: 1. 29   2. 08   3. Application
4. 5 = Implementation 5. Moderate

52. The nurse has instructed a 74-year-old client about his oral medications. The nurse determines that the client understands the instructions when the client says,

*A. "I shouldn't alter the dosage without contacting my doctor."
B. "If I miss a few of my hypertension medicines, I should take an extra one for a few days."
C. "If I should suddenly run out of my prescription, I can take an alternative medication."
D. "Medicines that are discolored can still be effective."

Reference: p. 662

Descriptors: 1. 29   2. 09   3. Application
4. 6 = Evaluation   5. Moderate

53. The nurse is caring for a 78-year-old client on several prescription medications who has limited financial resources. In teaching the client about the medications, the nurse should instruct the client to

A. ask the physician to prescribe brand-name drugs as they are cheaper.
B. avoid the use of over-the-counter drugs sold at discount stores.
*C. avoid borrowing from or loaning medications to other people.
D. explore the use of alternative therapies which may decrease drug dependence.

Reference: p. 662

Descriptors: 1. 29   2. 09   3. Application
             4. 5 = Implementation 5. Easy

CHAPTER 30
Perioperative Nursing

1. The nurse is caring for a perioperative client. The term "perioperative phase" refers to care given to a client

A. immediately before an operative procedure.
B. during the operative procedure.
C. immediately after an operative procedure.
*D. before, during, and after an operative procedure.

Reference: p. 670

Descriptors: 1. 30   2. 01   3. Factual
             4. 1 = No Process   5. Easy

2. The nurse is caring for a client who is scheduled for cardiac bypass surgery. The nurse should explain to the client and family that this type of surgery is classified as

A. minor.
*B. major.
C. elective.
D. constructive.

Reference: pp. 670–671

Descriptors: 1. 30   2. 01   3. Factual
             4. 5 = Implementation 5. Easy

3. The nurse is caring for a client scheduled for an appendectomy. The nurse should explain to the client that this type of procedure is termed

*A. ablative.
B. diagnostic.
C. therapeutic.
D. reconstructive.

Reference: p. 671

Descriptors: 1. 30   2. 01   3. Application
             4. 5 = Implementation 5. Easy

4. The nurse is caring for a client who will receive general anesthesia. The nurse should explain to the client that general anesthesia

A. is administered through the intravenous route.
B. allows the client to remain awake but unaware of the surgical procedure.
C. is often used for brief surgical procedures.
*D. can produce central nervous system depression.

Reference: p. 672

Descriptors: 1. 30   2. 01   3. Application
             4. 5 = Implementation 5. Moderate

5. A client is scheduled for a cesarean section delivery under spinal anesthesia. The nurse determines that the client understands the instructions given by the anesthesiologist when the client says,

A. "This type of anesthesia injects a local anesthetic around a nerve trunk."
B. "Central nervous system depression is a common side effect."
*C. "Following the surgery I may have a headache."
D. "My blood pressure may be elevated after the anesthesia is given."

Reference: p. 672

Descriptors: 1. 30   2. 01   3. Application
             4. 6 = Evaluation   5. Moderate

6. An adult client has signed an informed consent for surgery. One hour before surgery, the nurse offers the client a pre-operative medication. When the client asks the nurse "Why am I getting a pre-operative medication?"The nurse should

A. tell the client that the medication will help her to relax before surgery.
*B. explain the purpose of the medication, and if confusion continues, notify the physician.
C. cancel the client's surgery until the physician can explain to the client why surgery is necessary.
D. withhold the medication until the client can explain why surgery is necessary.

Reference: p. 672

Descriptors: 1. 30   2. 01   3. Application
             4. 5 = Implementation 5. Easy

7. An adult client is scheduled for outpatient surgery on her left wrist in two days. The nurse determines that the client needs *further* preoperative instructions when the client says,

   A. "I shouldn't wear any makeup or nail polish on the day of the surgery."
   B. "If possible, I should wear short-sleeve clothes that button down the front."
   C. "I should have someone available to drive me to my home after the procedure."
   *D. "It's acceptable to wear my watch and wedding rings as I usually do."

   Reference: p. 673

   Descriptors: 1. 30   2. 01   3. Application
                4. 6 = Evaluation   5. Moderate

8. An adult client with chronic obstructive pulmonary disease (COPD) is scheduled for surgery. Due to the client's medical history, the nurse should assess the client during the postoperative period for symptoms of

   A. hypoglycemia.
   B. hypotension.
   C. prolonged healing.
   *D. pneumonia.

   Reference: p. 675

   Descriptors: 1. 30   2. 02   3. Application
                4. 2 = Assessment   5. Easy

9. An adult client with diabetes mellitus is scheduled for a total hip replacement. Following the surgery, the nurse should give priority to assessing the client's

   *A. degree of wound healing.
   B. serum calcium level.
   C. degree of respiratory depression.
   D. ability to consume a regular diet.

   Reference: p. 675

   Descriptors: 1. 30   2. 02   3. Application
                4. 2 = Assessment   5. Moderate

10. An adult client scheduled for partial removal of a lung tells the nurse that he has been taking diuretics for the past year for hypertension. Following the surgery a priority assessment for the nurse to make is the client's

    A. degree of wound healing.
    B. blood glucose level.
    C. weight loss.
    *D. serum potassium level.

    Reference: p. 675

    Descriptors: 1. 30   2. 02   3. Application
                 4. 2 = Assessment   5. Moderate

11. The nurse is caring for an obese adult client in a home setting one week after knee replacement surgery. A priority nursing diagnosis for this client is

    *A. risk for infection related to client's obesity.
    B. altered nutrition: less than body requirements related to surgical procedure.
    C. anxiety related to pain and immobility as a result of surgery.
    D. knowledge deficit related to pain management techniques.

    Reference: p. 676

    Descriptors: 1. 30   2. 02   3. Application
                 4. 3 = Analysis/Diag.   5. Moderate

12. The nurse is caring for a client on the first postoperative day following abdominal surgery. The client has smoked one pack of cigarettes a day for 15 years. A priority assessment for the nurse to make is the client's

    A. cardiovascular sounds.
    B. ability to ambulate.
    C. nutritional status.
    *D. breath sounds.

    Reference: p. 676

    Descriptors: 1. 30   2. 02   3. Application
                 4. 2 = Assessment   5. Easy

13. An Asian-American client tells the nurse that she does not think she should ambulate to the chair on the first postoperative day following foot surgery. The nurse should

    A. ask the client's family member to encourage the client to ambulate.
    B. tell the client that the doctor has ordered her to get out of bed.
    C. inform the client that the nurse will return later and help her to the chair.
    *D. instruct the client about the reasons for early ambulation for postoperative care.

    Reference: p. 678

    Descriptors: 1. 30   2. 03   3. Application
                 4. 5 = Implementation   5. Moderate

14. An Asian-American adult client is scheduled to have a temporary colostomy to relieve a bowel obstruction. The client tells the nurse that she wants the colostomy only if it is truly temporary. A priority nursing diagnosis for this client is

    A. risk for infection related to extensive abdominal manipulation.
    B. ineffective airway clearance related to decreased breath sounds.
    *C. anticipatory grieving related to body image disturbance.
    D. ineffective individual coping related to conflict between need for surgery and cultural beliefs.

    Reference: p. 676

    Descriptors: 1. 30   2. 02   3. Application
                 4. 3 = Analysis/Diag.   5. Moderate

15. An adult client is scheduled for back surgery to repair a herniated disk. An important preoperative teaching plan for the nurse to make for this client should include

   A. nutritional needs following surgery.
   *B. ambulation from the bed to the chair.
   C. methods to prevent infection.
   D. use of blood transfusion equipment.

   Reference: p. 680

   Descriptors: 1. 30   2. 03   3. Application
                4. 4 = Planning   5. Moderate

16. A client is scheduled for a tubal ligation procedure. Before the client is taken to the surgical area, the nurse documents the client's vital signs. The nurse should explain to the client that this provides

   *A. baseline data for comparison during and after the procedure.
   B. routine data required of all clients scheduled for surgery.
   C. data which are useful for determining the type of anesthesia needed.
   D. data which can be used to determine how to position the client during the procedure.

   Reference: pp. 681, 685

   Descriptors: 1. 30   2. 04   3. Application
                4. 5 = Implementation 5. Moderate

17. The nurse is providing preoperative teaching for an 8-year-old client and his family. The child is scheduled for reconstructive surgery. To help alleviate the child's anxiety, the nurse plans to

   A. show the child a blood-pressure cuff.
   B. demonstrate how the patient-controlled analgesia machine is operated.
   C. have the child meet with the surgeon who will perform the procedure.
   *D. take the child and family on a tour of the operating room.

   Reference: p. 682

   Descriptors: 1. 30   2. 04   3. Application
                4. 4 = Planning   5. Easy

18. An adult client is scheduled for an appendectomy and general anesthesia with an endotracheal tube. The nurse should instruct the client that following the surgery, he may experience a

   *A. sore throat.
   B. gradual return of feeling in his throat.
   C. sensation of dizziness.
   D. feeling of abdominal fullness.

   Reference: p. 683

   Descriptors: 1. 30   2. 04   3. Application
                4. 5 = Implementation 5. Easy

19. Before surgery, the nurse has instructed a preoperative adult client about the use of pain medication following surgery. The nurse determines that the client needs *further* instructions when the client says,

   A. "I should ask for the pain medication before the pain gets severe."
   B. "If I can't have any food or water on the first day, I'll get pain medicine by injection."
   C. "If I use relaxation techniques, the pain medication will be more effective."
   * D. "I should wait until the pain becomes severe before requesting pain medication."

   Reference: p. 683

   Descriptors: 1. 30   2. 04   3. Application
                4. 6 = Evaluation   5. Moderate

20. The nurse is planning to instruct a client who will be undergoing abdominal surgery about postoperative deep breathing techniques. Which of the following should be included in the nurse's teaching plan?

   A. The exercises will be done every 4 hours for the first 24 to 48 hours after surgery.
   B. During the exercise the client should hold his breath and count to ten.
   C. The client should be sitting upright in a chair for the most effectiveness.
   *D. The client should be in a semi-Fowler's position with the head and shoulders supported.

   Reference: p. 683

   Descriptors: 1. 30   2. 04   3. Application
                4. 4 = Planning   5. Moderate

21. The nurse is assisting a client with coughing exercises on the first postoperative day. The nurse should

   *A. offer the client pain medication prior to the coughing exercises.
   B. have the client repeat the exercise every 4 hours during the first 24 hours after surgery.
   C. place the client in a side-lying position with a supportive pillow.
   D. instruct the client to take a deep breath and hold it for 10 seconds.

   Reference: p. 684

   Descriptors: 1. 30   2. 04   3. Application
                4. 5 = Implementation 5. Moderate

22. The nurse has instructed a client about incentive spirometry following surgery. The nurse determines that the client understands the instructions when the client says that incentive spirometry

   *A. is used to help increase lung volume.
   B. should be done while flat in bed.
   C. is performed once a day after surgery.
   D. can be done immediately after mealtime.

   Reference: p. 684

   Descriptors: 1. 30   2. 04   3. Application
                       4. 6 = Evaluation   5. Moderate

23. The nurse is planning to instruct an adult client who will be undergoing major surgery about leg exercises. The nurse should instruct the client that leg exercises

   A. need to be performed at least once per day.
   *B. help promote venous return.
   C. are important to prevent contractures.
   D. can improve respiratory function.

   Reference: p. 684

   Descriptors: 1. 30   2. 04   3. Application
                       4. 5 = Implementation 5. Easy

24. An adult client is scheduled for outpatient surgery to remove a mole on her forearm. The nurse should instruct the client that

   A. the forearm will be cleansed with Betadine by the surgeon.
   B. a shampoo is not necessary.
   C. the skin around the area should be shaved 24 hours before surgery.
   *D. the site should be cleansed with an antibacterial soap before surgery.

   Reference: p. 685

   Descriptors: 1. 30   2. 04   3. Application
                       4. 5 = Implementation 5. Moderate

25. An adult client who has had preoperative barium diagnostic tests has an order for an enema prior to surgery. The nurse plans to instruct the client that the purpose of the enema is to

   A. decrease straining during the postoperative period.
   *B. prevent constipation during the postoperative period.
   C. cleanse the bowel of all bacteria and feces.
   D. decrease the need for bowel elimination following surgery.

   Reference: p. 685

   Descriptors: 1. 30   2. 04   3. Application
                       4. 4 = Planning   5. Moderate

26. The nurse is caring for a 15-year-old client with a hearing aid a few hours before scheduled surgery on his knee. The nurse completing the preoperative checklist should

   A. omit asking about dentures.
   B. remove the client's hearing aid.
   C. place any jewelry on the bedside table.
   *D. leave the hearing aid in place.

   Reference: p. 686

   Descriptors: 1. 30   2. 04   3. Application
                       4. 5 = Implementation 5. Moderate

27. The nurse has given a preoperative client Demerol 100 mg IM an hour before surgery. The nurse plans to

   A. review the preoperative instructions one more time.
   B. assist the client to ambulate to the bathroom to void.
   *C. raise both siderails on the client's bed.
   D. complete the remainder of the preoperative checklist.

   Reference: p. 686

   Descriptors: 1. 30   2. 04   3. Application
                       4. 5 = Implementation 5. Moderate

28. The operating room nurse has just received a client in the holding area prior to surgery. A priority assessment for the nurse to make prior to surgery is to

   A. ask the client about any allergies.
   *B. identify the client by checking the identification band.
   C. determine whether family members are present.
   D. discuss any spiritual concerns the client may present.

   Reference: p. 687

   Descriptors: 1. 30   2. 07   3. Application
                       4. 5 = Implementation 5. Moderate

29. One of the primary responsibilities of the circulating nurse during the intraoperative phase is to ensure that the client's

   *A. physical safety is maintained.
   B. drapes are applied properly.
   C. surgical instruments remain sterile.
   D. anesthesia level is appropriate.

   Reference: p. 687

   Descriptors: 1. 30   2. 07   3. Application
                       4. 5 = Implementation 5. Moderate

30. A client is scheduled for a surgical procedure which requires that she be placed in a Trendelenburg position. Following the return of the client to the supine position the nurse should assess the client for

   *A. hypotension.
   B. hypertension.
   C. headache.
   D. back pain.

Reference: p. 688

Descriptors: 1. 30   2. 07   3. Application
            4. 2 = Assessment   5. Moderate

31. One hour after abdominal surgery with general anesthesia, the nurse observes that the client's pulse has increased from 80 beats per minute to 120 beats per minute and the client appears restless. The nurse should

   A. continue to monitor the client every 15 minutes.
   B. increase the intravenous fluid rate.
   C. assess the client's skin temperature.
   *D. notify the client's physician of the change in status.

Reference: p. 688

Descriptors: 1. 30   2. 05   3. Application
            4. 5 = Implementation 5. Moderate

32. Thirty minutes after abdominal surgery, the recovery room nurse determines that a client's pulse has increased from 68 beats per minute to 110 beats per minute and the client's skin is cool to the touch. The nurse notifies the client's physician as these symptoms are indicative of

   A. respiratory arrest.
   B. overmedication of anesthesia.
   *C. cardiovascular shock.
   D. fluid overload.

Reference: p. 689

Descriptors: 1. 30   2. 05   3. Application
            4. 3 = Analysis/Diag.   5. Moderate

33. During the recovery period following abdominal surgery the nurse determines that the client is still not fully conscious. The nurse plans to position the client in a

   A. prone position.
   B. supine position.
   C. semi-Fowler's position.
   *D. side-lying position.

Reference: p. 690

Descriptors: 1. 30   2. 06   3. Application
            4. 5 = Implementation 5. Moderate

34. The nurse is caring for an adult client who has had surgery to re-attach his left finger which was severed as a result of a farm accident. A priority diagnosis for this client in the recovery period is

   A. potential complication: thrombophlebitis related to surgery.
   *B. risk for infection related to traumatic wound of left finger in farm accident.
   C. impaired physical mobility related to traumatic wound surgery.
   D. body image disturbance related to potential loss of left finger.

Reference: p. 690

Descriptors: 1. 30   2. 06   3. Application
            4. 3 = Analysis/Diag.   5. Moderate

35. The nurse is caring for a client who has just been admitted to the hospital unit from the recovery room following surgery to remove a bullet from his left shoulder. The client asks for pain medication which has been ordered PRN every 3 to 4 hours. Before administering the pain medication the nurse should

   A. ask the client if he received any pain medication earlier.
   B. determine if the medication is really needed.
   C. evaluate the type of anesthesia that was given during surgery.
   *D. check the client's record to verify if analgesia was administered earlier.

Reference: p. 691

Descriptors: 1. 30   2. 06   3. Application
            4. 5 = Implementation 5. Moderate

36. While caring for a an adult client on the first postoperative day following a cesarean section delivery, to prevent thrombophlebitis the nurse should

   A. keep the client's legs elevated while in bed.
   *B. encourage the client to ambulate in the room.
   C. place two pillows under the client's knees.
   D. be certain that the antiembolic stockings are in place continuously.

Reference: p. 694

Descriptors: 1. 30   2. 07   3. Application
            4. 5 = Implementation 5. Moderate

37. The nurse determines that a postoperative client is experiencing hypovolemic shock. The nurse ensures that the client has a patent airway and then

   A. contacts the client's physician.
   B. places the client in Trendelenburg position.
   C. obtains an order for a type and crossmatch for blood.
   *D. elevates the client's legs 45°.

Reference: p. 694

Descriptors: 1. 30   2. 07   3. Application
            4. 5 = Implementation 5. Moderate

38. The nurse has provided a postoperative client with home care instructions prior to discharge. The nurse determines that the client understands the instructions about his care when he says,

*A. "If I have pain or redness in my calf, I should contact my physician."
B. "If thrombophlebitis develops, I will need to apply ice to the area."
C. "I should change my antiembolic stockings before I go to bed."
D. "If I develop a reddened area on my calf, massaging it will alleviate the pain."

Reference: pp. 694–695

Descriptors: 1. 30   2. 07   3. Application
            4. 6 = Evaluation   5. Moderate

39. While assessing a 2-day postoperative client, the client tells the nurse that he has had difficulty breathing and chest pain. The client's pulse is 124 beats per minute. The nurse should *first*

A. place the client in a high-Fowler's position.
B. increase the intravenous fluid rate.
*C. notify the physician immediately.
D. monitor the client's blood pressure.

Reference: p. 696

Descriptors: 1. 30   2. 07   3. Application
            4. 5 = Implementation 5. Moderate

40. While assessing a 78-year-old client who had a total hip replacement 3 days ago, the nurse observes that the client has a temperature of 100.6°F, purulent sputum, and lung crackles. The nurse determines that the client is most likely experiencing

A. tuberculosis.
B. atelectasis.
C. pulmonary embolism.
*D. pneumonia.

Reference: p. 696

Descriptors: 1. 30   2. 07   3. Interpretive
            4. 3 = Analysis/Diag.   5. Moderate

41. The nurse has auscultated the abdomen of a 4-day postoperative client and detects a high-pitched sound. The client tells the nurse that he has "a lot of abdominal distention." The nurse determines that the client is most likely experiencing

*A. paralytic ileus.
B. peristalsis.
C. flatus.
D. constipation.

Reference: p. 696

Descriptors: 1. 30   2. 07   3. Interpretive
            4. 3 = Analysis/Diag.   5. Moderate

42. The nurse visits a client in the home on the second postoperative day. The client tells the nurse she has had "a lot of hiccups and can't seem to get rid of them." The nurse should instruct the client to

A. chew some ice chips.
B. drink several glasses of water.
C. eat a teaspoon of salt.
*D. rebreathe into a paper bag.

Reference: p. 697

Descriptors: 1. 30   2. 11   3. Application
            4. 5 = Implementation 5. Moderate

43. A young mother visits the Urgent Care Center because her 12-year-old son fell and bruised his knee. The wound is closed and bruised and the child complains of pain and swelling. The nurse should instruct the mother that this type of wound is termed a/an

A. laceration.
*B. contusion.
C. abrasion.
D. inflammation.

Reference: p. 696

Descriptors: 1. 30   2. 08   3. Application
            4. 5 = Implementation 5. Moderate

44. The nurse makes a home visit to a 79-year-old client who had a total knee replacement 1 week ago. To promote wound healing, the nurse should instruct the client to consume foods which are high in

A. potassium.
B. vitamin D.
*C. vitamin C.
D. calcium.

Reference: p. 700

Descriptors: 1. 30   2. 09   3. Application
            4. 5 = Implementation 5. Moderate

45. While changing a homebound client's dressing following a mastectomy, the nurse notes a clear watery drainage. The nurse documents this drainage as

A. purulent.
B. sanguineous.
C. serosanguineous.
*D. serous.

Reference: p. 702

Descriptors: 1. 30   2. 10   3. Application
            4. 5 = Implementation 5. Moderate

46. The nurse changes a home care client's dressing over his abdominal incision on the seventh post-operative day and notes excessive amounts of serosanguineous fluid on the wound and dressing. The nurse determines that the client is most likely experiencing

A. wound infection.
B. normal wound healing.
*C. impending dehiscence.
D. total eviceration.

Reference: p. 703

Descriptors: 1. 30   2. 09   3. Interpretive
            4. 3 = Analysis/Diag.   5. Moderate

47. A frantic mother enters the emergency room of a local hospital with her child and tells the nurse that her 10-year-old has been bitten on her finger by a stray dog. After assessing the puncture wound, the nurse should *first*

A. flush the wound with normal saline.
*B. assess when the last tetanus shot was given.
C. hold the wound edges together with tape.
D. cover the wound with a light dressing.

Reference: pp. 704–705

Descriptors: 1. 30   2. 09   3. Application
            4. 5 = Implementation 5. Moderate

48. The nurse has instructed an adult client how to change her dressings at home. During a return demonstration of the dressing change, the nurse determines that the client has understood the instructions when the nurse observes the client

*A. don sterile gloves after pouring the cleaning solution.
B. don sterile gloves to remove the old dressing.
C. cleanse the wound from the edges inward toward center.
D. use one moistened gauze square for the entire dressing change.

Reference: pp. 710–711

Descriptors: 1. 30   2. 11   3. Application
            4. 6 = Evaluation   5. Moderate

49. The nurse is preparing to apply a roller bandage to a client's leg which was amputated at the knee. An appropriate turn for the nurse to use for this bandage is the

A. spica.
B. figure-of-eight.
C. spiral reverse.
*D. recurrent.

Reference: pp. 713, 715

Descriptors: 1. 30   2. 07   3. Application
            4. 5 = Implementation 5. Moderate

50. The nurse has instructed a family member how to irrigate a client's wound with normal saline. During the return demonstration the nurse determines that the family member needs *further* instructions when the nurse observes the caregiver

A. use warmed normal saline.
B. flush the wound until clear.
*C. don sterile gloves to remove the old dressing.
D. pack the wound loosely with gauze.

Reference: pp. 719–720

Descriptors: 1. 30   2. 11   3. Application
            4. 6 = Evaluation   5. Moderate

UNIT VII
PROMOTING HEALTHY PSYCHOSOCIAL RESPONSES

CHAPTER 31
Self-Concept

1. A client who recently lost 100 pounds continues to shop for clothes in her "old size." This is an example of a disruption of

   A. body image.
   *B. subjective self.
   C. ideal self.
   D. social self.

   Reference: p. 729

   Descriptors: 1. 31   2. 01   3. Application
               4. 3 = Analysis/Diag.   5. Easy

2. The question "Are you able to look at yourself in the mirror and like what you see?" is asking about which dimension of self-concept?

   A. Self-concept
   B. Self-expectation
   *C. Self-evaluation
   D. Self-orientation

   Reference: pp. 729–730

   Descriptors: 1. 31   2. 02   3. Application
               4. 1 = No Process   5. Moderate

3. An overweight client experiencing low self-esteem may be having difficulties with which step in the formation of self-concept?

   *A. Positive separation of self from the environment
   B. Externalization of other people's attitude towards self
   C. Internalization of societal standards
   D. Rejection of societal standards

   Reference: pp. 730–731

   Descriptors: 1. 31   2. 03   3. Application
               4. 3 = Analysis/Diag.   5. Moderate

4. When counseling a client on factors that affect self-concept, which of the following statements denotes a possible misunderstanding?

   A. "Having a good job means a lot to me."
   B. "My parents instilled strong beliefs in me."
   C. "It's important to me to be the best in all I do."
   *D. "My Hispanic background doesn't affect anything about me."

   Reference: pp. 731–733

   Descriptors: 1. 31   2. 05   3. Interpretive
               4. 6 = Evaluation   5. Moderate

5. A client is unable to describe himself in any positive way and accentuates his weaknesses. A possible nursing diagnosis can be based upon the client's

   A. positive self-concept.
   *B. negative self-concept.
   C. high self-esteem.
   D. low self-esteem.

   Reference: pp. 736–741

   Descriptors: 1. 31   2. 04, 07   3. Application
               4. 3 = Analysis/Diag.   5. Moderate

6. When assessing the possible impact a mastectomy may have on the client, an appropriate comment is

   *A. "Can you tell me how this surgery will change the way you feel about yourself?"
   B. "Your breasts are important to you, aren't they?"
   C. "Why are you so concerned with your appearance?"
   D. "Tell me about your illness."

   Reference: pp. 734–735

   Descriptors: 1. 31   2. 06   3. Application
               4. 2 = Assessment   5. Moderate

7. An appropriate question when assessing a client's self-expectations about weight loss is

   A. "What makes you think you can change your eating habits?"
   B. "How do you feel about losing weight?"
   C. "How important is it that you lose weight?"
   *D. "What do you think is a realistic weekly weight loss for you?"

   Reference: pp. 734–735

   Descriptors: 1. 31   2. 06   3. Application
               4. 2 = Assessment   5. Moderate

8. A client who recently lost 50 pounds just received news that she is pregnant. A possible nursing diagnosis is

   A. actual chronic low self-esteem related to obesity.
   B. potential chronic low self-esteem related to obesity.
   C. actual situational low self-esteem related to fear of weight regain and pregnancy.
   *D. potential situational low self-esteem related to fear of weight regain and pregnancy.

   Reference: pp. 737–740

   Descriptors: 1. 31   2. 07   3. Application
               4. 3 = Analysis/Diag.   5. Moderate

9. The most effective nursing strategy to assist a client in recognizing and using personal strength includes

*A. encouraging the client's self-identification of strengths.
  B. promoting the client's active external thinking.
  C. listening to the client and providing advice as needed.
  D. assisting the client in mainatining an external locus of control.

Reference: pp. 741–743

Descriptors: 1. 31   2. 08   3. Application
              4. 5 = Implementation 5. Moderate

10. Appropriate nursing strategies to assist a client in maintaining a sense of self include

  A. using the client's first name when addressing the client.
*B. treating the client with dignity.
  C. explaining procedures only if the client is attentive.
  D. discouraging the use of personal items.

Reference: pp. 741–743

Descriptors: 1. 31   2. 08   3. Application
              4. 5 = Implementation 5. Moderate

11. A successful resolution of the nursing diagnosis "Negative self-concept related to unrealistic self-expectations" is when the client can

  A. report a positive self-concept.
  B. identify negative thoughts.
*C. recognize positive thoughts.
  D. give one positive cue with each negative cue.

Reference: pp. 743–744

Descriptors: 1. 31   2. 09   3. Application
              4. 6 = Evaluation 5. Difficult

CHAPTER 32
Stress and Adaptation

1. The change that takes place in human beings as a response to a stressor is termed

  A. homostasis.
  B. reaction.
*C. adaptation.
  D. reorganization.

Reference: p. 755

Descriptors: 1. 32   2. 03   3. Factual
              4. 1 = No Process 5. Easy

2. In human beings, the fight-or-flight response is controlled by the

  A. pituitary gland.
  B. adrenal gland.
  C. parasympathetic nervous system.
*D. sympathetic nervous system.

Reference: p. 757

Descriptors: 1. 32   2. 02   3. Factual
              4. 1 = No Process 5. Easy

3. When a child touches a hot burner on a stove, the first localized response to the body is the

*A. reflex pain response.
  B. inflammatory response.
  C. alarm reaction.
  D. shock reaction.

Reference: p. 758

Descriptors: 1. 32   2. 02   3. Factual
              4. 1 = No Process 5. Easy

4. In the general adaptation syndrome the phase in which the body has an increase in energy levels and increased cardiac output is the

  A. resistance phase.
  B. exhaustion phase.
*C. shock phase.
  D. reaction phase.

Reference: p. 758

Descriptors: 1. 32   2. 05   3. Factual
              4. 1 = No Process 5. Easy

5. Various forms of anxiety have different effects on human beings. The type of anxiety which serves to increase motivation and facilitate problem-solving is

*A. mild anxiety.
  B. moderate anxiety.
  C. severe anxiety.
  D. fearful anxiety.

Reference: pp. 759–760

Descriptors: 1. 32   2. 04   3. Factual
              4. 1 = No Process 5. Easy

6. The wife of a hospitalized client with terminal cancer tells the nurse that she doesn't visit her husband very often because she just cannot deal with the fact that he is dying. The nurse determines that the client's wife is demonstrating a behavior termed

  A. compromise.
  B. repression.
*C. withdrawal.
  D. suppression.

Reference: p. 760

Descriptors: 1. 32   2. 05   3. Application
              4. 2 = Assessment 5. Easy

7. After caring for an angry hospitalized client, the nurse enters the nurse's station and throws the client's chart onto the desk. The nurse is demonstrating a defense mechanism termed

   A. reaction formation.
   *B. displacement.
   C. regression.
   D. suppression.

   Reference: p. 780

   Descriptors: 1. 32   2. 05   3. Application
                       4. 2 = Assessment   5. Moderate

8. The nurse is caring for a 3-year-old child hospitalized for cardiac surgery. The child was toilet-trained but has begun to soil the bed linens. The nurse determines that the child is demonstrating a defense mechanism termed

   *A. regression.
   B. repression.
   C. projection.
   D. sublimation.

   Reference: p. 760

   Descriptors: 1. 32   2. 05   3. Application
                       4. 2 = Assessment   5. Easy

9. A client with hypertension visits the clinic for his annual check-up when he tells the nurse he has been working 80 hours a week to establish his own business. The nurse determines that the client's stress is related to the basic human need of

   A. love and belonging.
   B. safety and security.
   C. self-actualization.
   *D. self-esteem.

   Reference: p. 761

   Descriptors: 1. 32   2. 06   3. Application
                       4. 2 = Assessment   5. Moderate

10. The nurse makes a home visit to a family where the adult male has Alzheimer's disease. The client's wife is the primary caregiver and tells the nurse that she is exhausted from caring for her deteriorating husband. The nurse determines that the wife is experiencing

    A. role strain.
    B. situational crisis.
    C. caregiver burnout.
    *D. caregiver burden.

    Reference: p. 763

    Descriptors: 1. 32   2. 06   3. Application
                        4. 3 = Analysis/Diag.   5. Moderate

11. A client visits the clinic and the nurse determines that she is approximately 10 weeks pregnant. She tells the nurse that the pregnancy was not planned and she doesn't know if her husband wants a baby right now. The nurse determines that the client is experiencing

    A. developmental crisis.
    B. anticipatory stress.
    *C. situational stress.
    D. moderate anxiety.

    Reference: p. 764

    Descriptors: 1. 32   2. 01   3. Application
                        4. 3 = Analysis/Diag.   5. Moderate

12. The nurse is caring for a family in the community that is experiencing stress related to the primary wage earner being laid off from his job. The wife tells the nurse that her husband hasn't been sleeping well at night. A priority nursing diagnosis for this family is

    A. hopelessness related to inability to find work.
    *B. defensive coping related to loss of employment.
    C. decisional conflict related to anxiety.
    D. situational distress related to financial concerns.

    Reference: p. 766

    Descriptors: 1. 32   2. 05   3. Application
                        4. 3 = Analysis/Diag.   5. Moderate

13. The nurse is caring for an obese 20-year-old client who tells the nurse that she "has always been fat and hates diet foods." A priority nursing diagnosis for this client is

    A. individual coping, potential for growth.
    B. denial related to being overweight.
    *C. defensive coping related to long-term obesity.
    D. ineffective denial related to poor nutritional status.

    Reference: p. 767

    Descriptors: 1. 32   2. 05   3. Application
                        4. 3 = Analysis/Diag.   5. Moderate

14. The nurse is caring for an expectant mother who expresses fears about parenting. The nurse should suggest a stress management technique termed

    A. meditation.
    *B. anticipatory socialization.
    C. crisis intervention.
    D. progressive muscle relaxation.

    Reference: p. 770

    Descriptors: 1. 32   2. 07   3. Application
                        4. 5 = Implementation 5. Moderate

15. The nurse has been working with a family by using crisis intervention techniques. The nurse is concluding her care with the family and asks the family to complete the final step of the process. The nurse should ask the family to

A. identify alternatives.
B. choose from among the alternatives.
C. accept what they cannot change.
*D. evaluate the outcomes.

Reference: p. 772

Descriptors: 1. 32   2. 07   3. Application
4. 5 = Implementation 5. Moderate

16. A nurse employed in an intensive care unit of a hospital finds that the job is very stressful. An appropriate stress management activity for the nurse to engage in is to

*A. become involved in constructive change.
B. sleep 4 to 6 hours every night.
C. exercise for 20 minutes once a week.
D. eat high-carbohydrate foods daily.

Reference: p. 773

Descriptors: 1. 32   2. 08   3. Application
4. 5 = Implementation 5. Moderate

CHAPTER 33
Loss, Grief, and Death

1. The daughter of a hospitalized client who is dying has been crying outside of her father's room. The nurse determines that the daughter is experiencing a/an

A. actual loss.
B. perceived loss.
C. personal loss.
*D. anticipatory loss.

Reference: p. 781

Descriptors: 1. 33   2. 02   3. Application
4. 3 = Analysis/Diag.   5. Easy

2. A 78-year-old client tells the nurse that she hasn't been eating very well since the loss of her husband 2 months ago. The nurse determines that the client is in a state of

A. shock.
B. mourning.
*C. bereavement.
D. acceptance.

Reference: pp. 781–782

Descriptors: 1. 33   2. 03   3. Application
4. 3 = Analysis/Diag.   5. Moderate

3. A hospitalized client has just been informed that he has terminal cancer. He says to the nurse, "There must be some mistake in the diagnosis." The nurse determines that the client is demonstrating which of the following?

*A. Denial
B. Anger
C. Bargaining
D. Acceptance

Reference: p. 782

Descriptors: 1. 33   2. 04   3. Application
4. 2 = Assessment   5. Easy

4. The nurse is caring for a client who is dying of terminal cancer. While assessing the client for signs of impending death, the nurse should observe the client for

A. elevated blood pressure.
*B. Cheyne-Stokes respirations.
C. elevated pulse rate.
D. decreased temperature.

Reference: p. 784

Descriptors: 1. 33   2. 11   3. Application
4. 2 = Assessment   5. Moderate

5. In the United States, several definitions of death are currently being used. The definition which uses apnea testing and pupillary responses to light is termed

*A. whole brain death.
B. heart-lung death.
C. circulatory death.
D. higher brain death.

Reference: p. 784

Descriptors: 1. 33   2. 05   3. Factual
4. 1 = No Process   5. Moderate

6. The nurse is caring for a dying client who has persistently requested that the nurse "help her to die and be in peace." According to the Code for Nurses, the nurse should

A. ask the client if she has signed the advance directives document.
B. tell the client that the nurse will ask another nurse to care for the client.
C. instruct the client that only a physician can legally assist a suicide.
*D. try to make the client as comfortable as possible but refuse to assist in the death.

Reference: pp. 789–790

Descriptors: 1. 33   2. 10   3. Application
4. 5 = Implementation 5. Moderate

7. The nurse is caring for a terminally ill client when the physician tells the nurse that if necessary, only a "slow-code" should be initiated for the client. The nurse should

   *A. ask the physician to write do-not-resuscitate orders for the client.
   B. ask the family if this is the client's desire.
   C. instruct the cardiopulmonary resuscitation team that a "slow-code" has been ordered.
   D. tell the client that his life will not be prolonged indefinitely.

   Reference: p. 790

   Descriptors: 1. 33   2. 06   3. Application
   4. 5 = Implementation 5. Moderate

8. A physician writes orders for a client who has experienced brain death to have terminal weaning. The nurse plans to support the family members by

   A. informing them that this will result in inevitable death.
   B. providing them with analgesia during the process if necessary.
   *C. describing what to expect during the process.
   D. helping them to make funeral arrangements for the dying client.

   Reference: p. 791

   Descriptors: 1. 33   2. 08   3. Application
   4. 4 = Planning   5. Moderate

9. A client who is apparently dead is brought to the hospital by ambulance. The client was found alone in his apartment by a neighbor. Even though the family has refused an autopsy, an autopsy can be ordered by the

   A. family's physician.
   B. county court.
   C. city police department.
   *D. county coroner.

   Reference: p. 791

   Descriptors: 1. 33   2. 12   3. Factual
   4. 1 = No Process   5. Moderate

10. The nurse is caring for a 4-year-old client in the clinic when the mother expresses concerns about the child's toilet training. The child was toilet-trained completely but suffered the loss of her father in an auto accident 2 months ago. The nurse should explain to the mother that the child's behavior indicates a

    *A. normal grief response.
    B. dysfunctional grief response.
    C. need for psychological counseling.
    D. fear of her own death.

    Reference: p. 792

    Descriptors: 1. 33   2. 07   3. Application
    4. 3 = Analysis/Diag.   5. Moderate

11. The nurse is caring for a 70-year-old client who is receiving chemotherapy. The client requests pain medication every 2 hours. A priority nursing diagnosis for this client is

    A. anxiety related to fear of dying.
    *B. altered comfort related to effects of chemotherapy.
    C. fatigue related to heavy sedation.
    D. knowledge deficit related to effects of medications.

    Reference: p. 794

    Descriptors: 1. 33   2. 09   3. Application
    4. 3 = Analysis/Diag.   5. Moderate

12. The nurse has informed the family of a terminally ill comatose client about the loss of various senses during imminent death. The nurse determines that the family understands the instructions when one of the family members says that it is believed that the last sense to leave the body is the sense of

    A. taste.
    B. touch.
    C. smell.
    *D. hearing.

    Reference: p. 797

    Descriptors: 1. 33   2. 08   3. Application
    4. 6 = Evaluation   5. Moderate

13. Following the death of a terminally ill client, the nurse is legally responsible for

    A. washing the body thoroughly.
    B. removing any tubes in place.
    *C. identifying the body.
    D. requesting organ donations from the family.

    Reference: p. 802

    Descriptors: 1. 33   2. 12   3. Application
    4. 5 = Implementation 5. Moderate

14. The nurse in the Urgent Care clinic observes several family members behaving in a stunned manner after the physician has informed the family that their 16-month-old child is dead. The physician suspects that the child died of Sudden Infant Death Syndrome. The nurse should

    A. ask the family to make funeral arrangements.
    B. determine if the family is willing to make an organ donation.
    C. urge the family members to return home.
    *D. provide a quiet place for the family to grieve.

    Reference: p. 802

    Descriptors: 1. 33   2. 13   3. Application
    4. 5 = Implementation 5. Moderate

15. The nurse is caring for a competent 78-year-old client who is diagnosed with a terminal illness. After planning care with the client, an appropriate outcome is that the client will

A. demonstrate all phases of the grief process.
B. determine who will be with the client during the time of death.
*C. share concerns with significant others and seek needed help.
D. formulate plans for funeral arrangements following the death.

Reference: p. 803

Descriptors: 1. 33   2. 08   3. Application
            4. 4 = Planning   5. Moderate

CHAPTER 34
Sensory Stimulation

1. The ability to sit upright in a chair is due in part to which of the following types of sensory reception?

A. Visual
B. Tactile
*C. Kinesthetic
D. Musculoskeletal

Reference: p. 814

Descriptors: 1. 34   2. 01   3. Application
            4. 1 = No Process   5. Easy

2. An example of a complete sensory experience is

A. pin-skin-nerve-movement.
*B. flower-nose-olfactory nerve-rose.
C. heat-skin-nerve-blister.
D. food-tongue-hypoglossal-swallow.

Reference: p. 814

Descriptors: 1. 34   2. 02   3. Application
            4. 1 = No Process   5. Moderate

3. The purpose of the recticular activating system (RAS) in the sensory experience is to

A. alert people to more aesthetic situations.
B. force the body to recognize all stimuli.
*C. remember information not immediately acted upon.
D. maintain a sense of balance.

Reference: pp. 814–815

Descriptors: 1. 34   2. 03   3. Application
            4. 1 = No Process   5. Easy

4. Which of the following clients are most likely to experience sensory overload?

*A. A client who has spent 14 days in the Intensive Care Unit (ICU)
B. A prisoner in solitary confinement
C. A person who is blind and deaf
D. A client who has postoperative pain for three weeks

Reference: pp. 815–818

Descriptors: 1. 34   2. 01, 04   3. Interpretive
            4. 2 = Assessment   5. Moderate

5. Appropriate assessment data to collect when assessing a client's need for sensory stimulation include

A. weight.
*B. culture.
C. race.
D. gender.

Reference: pp. 818–819

Descriptors: 1. 34   2. 05   3. Application
            4. 2 = Assessment   5. Moderate

6. When a client is experiencing hand and wrist numbness, the nurse should conduct a

A. general nerve assessment.
B. cranial nerve sensory assessment.
C. cranial nerve motor assessment.
*D. peripheral nerve motor assesssment.

Reference: pp. 819–822

Descriptors: 1. 34   2. 05   3. Interpretive
            4. 2 = Assessment   5. Moderate

7. An appropriate nursing diagnosis for the client experiencing depression and boredom due to blindness is

A. altered sensory reception, integration, related to blindness.
B. impaired communication related to receiving and perceiving sensory stimuli.
*C. diversional activity deficit, related to impaired vision.
D. anxiety, related to paranoia stemming from impaired vision.

Reference: pp. 822–824

Descriptors: 1. 34   2. 06   3. Interpretive
            4. 3 = Analysis/Diag.   5. Difficult

8. Which of the following is not an appropriate nursing strategy to prevent sensory deprivation in the elderly client?

A. Determine need for glasses or a hearing aid.
B. Note fit and condition of dentures.
C. Provide large print books and magazines.
*D. Prescribe eye drops to assist in clearer vision.

Reference: pp. 825–829

Descriptors: 1. 34   2. 07   3. Interpretive
            4. 5 = implementation 5. Moderate

9. An appropriate nursing strategy to prevent sensory deprivation in an infant includes

 *A. talking to the infant when changing the diaper.
  B. limiting visual stimulation to reduce confusion.
  C. allowing the infant to crawl up and down stairs.
  D. providing mouth-sized toys for oral stimulation.

Reference: pp. 825–829

Descriptors: 1. 34   2. 07   3. Interpretive
             4. 5 = Implementation 5. Moderate

10. Successful resolution of the nursing diagnosis "Sleep pattern disturbance, related to sensory overload" is if the client

 *A. stated that a nap was restful.
  B. received a hypnotic.
  C. maintained a darkened, quiet environment.
  D. maintained bedtime rituals.

Reference: pp. 829–832

Descriptors: 1. 34   2. 08   3. Interpretive
             4. 6 = Evaluation   5. Moderate

11. In caring for clients who are deaf and blind, effective nursing strategies to prevent sensory deprivation include

  A. loud music to entertain client.
 *B. gentle touch before initiating care.
  C. sitting in front of the client when communicating.
  D. kinesthetic experiences such as dancing.

Reference: pp. 829–832

Descriptors: 1. 34   2. 07, 08 3. Application
             4. 5 = Implementation 5. Moderate

CHAPTER 35
Sexuality

1. The clitoris is similar to which male reproductive organ?

  A. Testis
 *B. Penis
  C. Scrotum
  D. Hymen

Reference: pp. 841–845

Descriptors: 1. 35   2. 01, 02 3. Application
             4. 1 = No Process   5. Easy

2. The major difference in the male and female physiologic sexual response is that

  A. males have a heightened excitement phase.
  B. males can only ejaculate during orgasm.
 *C. females experience no refractory period.
  D. females experience a less intense orgasmic phase.

Reference: pp. 845–846

Descriptors: 1. 35   2. 03   3. Interpretive
             4. 1 = No Process   5. Easy

3. For which of the following clients is obtaining a sexual history most important? A client with

  A. hypertension managed by diet.
 *B. impending colostomy surgery.
  C. active tuberculosis.
  D. pneumonia.

Reference: pp. 849–855

Descriptors: 1. 35   2. 04   3. Interpretive
             4. 2 = Assessment   5. Moderate

4. An appropriate question to ask when interviewing a client about satisfaction with their sexual expression is

  A. "Are you happy with your sex life?"
 *B. "If anything, what would you change about your sex life?"
  C. "Are you happy with your current partner?"
  D. "How's your sex life?"

Reference: pp. 857–860

Descriptors: 1. 35   2. 05   3. Interpretive
             4. 2 = Assessment   5. Moderate

5. Equipment necessary for a vaginal exam for sexually transmitted diseases (STD) include all of the following except

 *A. Pap smear slide.
  B. speculum.
  C. gloves.
  D. culture media.

Reference: pp. 860–861

Descriptors: 1. 35   2. 05, 09 3. Interpretive
             4. 4 = Planning   5. Moderate

6. When assessing a male client for erectile failure, the nurse should assess all of the following except:

  A. the use of anti-hypertensive medications.
  B. urinary elimination pattern.
  C. previous sexual activity.
 *D. allergies to environmental substances.

References: pp. 849–855

Descriptors: 1. 35   2. 05, 06 3. Interpretive
             4. 2 = Assessment   5. Difficult

7. An appropriate nursing diagnosis for the post-menopausal client experiencing dyspareunia is

A. pain, related to illness.
B. pain, related to the aging process.
C. altered sexuality pattern, related to the aging process.
*D. sexual dysfunction, related to postmenopausal symptoms.

Reference: pp. 861–862

Descriptors: 1. 35   2. 07   3. Interpretive
            4. 3 = Analysis/Diag.   5. Difficult

CHAPTER 36
Spirituality

1. The three universal spiritual needs include all of the following except

A. meaning and purpose.
B. love and relatedness.
C. forgiveness.
*D. God's permission.

Reference: p. 883

Descriptors: 1. 36   2. 02   3. Factual
            4. 1 = No Process   5. Easy

2. The difference between spirituality and religion is that spirituality is a/an

A. belief about a higher power.
*B. individual's relationship with a higher power.
C. organized worship.
D. belief in invisible energy or ideal.

Reference: pp. 883–884

Descriptors: 1. 36   2. 01, 06   3. Interpretive
            4. 1 = No Process   5. Moderate

3. Spirituality affects a client's life in all of the following areas except

A. nutritional intake.
B. ability to handle stress.
C. sexual expression.
*D. genetic makeup.

Reference: pp. 883–884

Descriptors: 1. 36   2. 03   3. Interpretive
            4. 2 = Assessment   5. Moderate

4. Which of the following is an example of a religious belief that is a life-denying experience?

A. Sacrament of the sick/Roman Catholic
B. Kosher foods/Jewish
*C. Restrictions on sterilization/Islam
D. Yoga and biofeedback/Middle East

Reference: pp. 885–888

Descriptors: 1. 36   2. 04, 05   3. Interpretive
            4. 3 = Analysis/Diag.   5. Moderate

5. Data for a spirituality assessment include

*A. general spiritual beliefs.
B. judgement about a client's beliefs.
C. parent's spiritual beliefs.
D. rationale for specific beliefs.

Reference: pp. 889–890

Descriptors: 1. 36   2. 07   3. Application
            4. 2 = Assessment   5. Moderate

6. An appropriate question to assess a client's specific spiritual needs during a hospital stay is

*A. "Do you have any spiritual or religious concerns that may affect your care?"
B. "What do you want from me to help you with your relationship with God?"
C. "Are you angry at God for letting you get sick?"
D. "What's your faith or religious affiliation?"

Reference: pp. 890–891

Descriptors: 1. 36   2. 07   3. Interpretive
            4. 2 = Assessment   5. Moderate

7. The client who expresses her spiritual anger to God for allowing her spouse to die is experiencing?

A. Spiritual distress: spousal loss, related to anger
*B. Spiritual distress: anger, related to spousal loss
C. Dysfunctional grieving, related to spousal loss
D. Hopelessness, related to spousal loss

Reference: p. 891

Descriptors: 1. 36   2. 08   3. Interpretive
            4. 3 = Analysis/Diag.   5. Difficult

8. Appropriate nursing action for the client goal "Develop and maintain positive spiritual practices" includes

A. noting the client's request to keep their rosary while in surgery.
B. judging the client's specific spiritual needs and requests.
*C. encouraging the attendance of the pastor at the client's bedside.
D. client states that he is at peace with his impending death.

Reference: pp. 891–896

Descriptors: 1. 36   2. 09   3. Interpretive
            4. 5 = Implementation 5. Moderate

9. A successful resolution of the nursing diagnosis "Spiritual distress, related to anger over spouse's death" is if the client

A. discusses his anger with the nurse.
*B. reconciles his anger with his higher power.
C. asks to go to the hospital chapel.
D. tells his daughter he is angry.

Reference: pp. 897–898

Descriptors: 1. 36   2. 10   3. Interpretive
            4. 6 = Evaluation   5. Moderate

UNIT VIII
PROMOTING HEALTHY
PHYSIOLOGIC RESPONSES

CHAPTER 37
Hygiene

1. While bathing an adult client, the nurse observes slight bruising on the client's forearm. The nurse plans to document this assessment of the client's integumentary system as

   A. sebaceous.
   *B. ecchymosis of the dermis.
   C. sebaceous cyst.
   D. epidermal abrasion.

   Reference: p. 911

   Descriptors: 1. 37   2. 01   3. Application
                4. 4 = Planning   5. Moderate

2. The nurse has presented a class on hygiene to a group of high school students. The nurse determines that one of the students needs *further* instructions when the student says that one of the primary functions of the skin is to

   *A. store iron.
   B. protect the body.
   C. excrete waste products.
   D. absorb vitamin D.

   Reference: p. 912

   Descriptors: 1. 37   2. 02   3. Application
                4. 6 = Evaluation   5. Moderate

3. The nurse is planning a presentation about hygiene and skin care to a group of adolescents. Which of the following would be important to include in the teaching plan?

   A. Average size individuals tend to be more susceptible to skin irritation as compared to obese individuals.
   B. As one ages, wrinkles may appear and are deep in the skin's epidermis.
   C. Adolescents tend to have skin which is dry and rough due to excessive outdoor exposure.
   *D. In the adolescent, enlarged sebaceous glands are due to hormonal changes in the body.

   Reference: p. 913

   Descriptors: 1. 37   2. 02   3. Application
                4. 4 = Planning   5. Moderate

4. A 63-year-old client in the clinic asks the nurse what she can do to get rid of the brown spots on her hands. The nurse should explain to the client that

   *A. she should avoid exposure to wind and sun.
   B. special handcreams are available by prescription to remove the spots.
   C. the physician should be notified as these may indicate liver disease.
   D. brown spots occur due to biliary blockage, so high-fat foods should be avoided.

   Reference: p. 913

   Descriptors: 1. 37   2. 02   3. Application
                4. 5 = Implementation 5. Moderate

5. An adult client from West Africa is hospitalized following abdominal surgery. On the second postoperative day, the client refuses a complete bath by the nurse. The nurse should

   A. tell the client that it is hospital policy that postoperative clients receive a daily bath.
   B. ask another nurse to assist in giving the client a complete bath.
   *C. negotiate with the client for a partial bath as his culture may influence his hygiene practices.
   D. contact the charge nurse and ask for advice on how to accomplish the bath with this client.

   Reference: p. 913

   Descriptors: 1. 37   2. 03   3. Application
                4. 5 = Implementation 5. Moderate

6. The nurse is caring for a 76-year-old client who is seen in the clinic because of dry, scaly skin. An appropriate question for the nurse to ask during the assessment of this client is

   *A. "Does the area cause itching?"
   B. "Do you find that you have more bruising?"
   C. "Is your skin warm to the touch?"
   D. "Have you noticed any moles on your skin?"

   Reference: pp. 914–915

   Descriptors: 1. 37   2. 03   3. Application
                4. 5 = Implementation 5. Moderate

7. An adult client has recently had bilateral bunionectomy surgery and has had difficulty maintaining her normal hygiene routine. A priority diagnosis for this client is

A. body image disturbance related to surgery.
B. impaired skin integrity related to poor circulation.
C. impaired social interaction related to immobility.
*D. self-care deficit related to immobility.

Reference: p. 916

Descriptors: 1. 37   2. 05   3. Interpretive
            4. 3 = Analysis/Diag.   5. Moderate

8. The nurse observes a small nodule on an adult client's left wrist while assisting the client with a bath. The nurse should *first*

A. document the finding in the client's record.
*B. compare the right wrist with the left wrist.
C. report the finding to the client's physician.
D. ask the client if the nodule is swollen.

Reference: p. 916

Descriptors: 1. 37   2. 04   3. Application
            4. 5 = Implementation 5. Moderate

9. The nurse is caring for a hospitalized client who is receiving intravenous chemotherapy. During every shift, the nurse should examine the client's

A. pressure points.
B. sensation of tempertures.
*C. infusion site.
D. skin elasticity.

Reference: p. 917

Descriptors: 1. 37   2. 09   3. Application
            4. 5 = Implementation 5. Moderate

10. The nurse is performing a physical assessment of a diabetic adult client's skin. The nurse pays particular attention to the client's skin for

*A. ulcerations.
B. macules.
C. rashes.
D. moles.

Reference: p. 917

Descriptors: 1. 37   2. 04   3. Application
            4. 2 = Assessment   5. Moderate

11. During morning report, the night nurse tells the oncoming nurse that an adult client is able to have a partial bath. The nurse plans to assist the client with bathing the

A. face.
B. arms.
C. chest.
*D. back.

Reference: p. 918

Descriptors: 1. 37   2. 06   3. Application
            4. 4 = Planning   5. Easy

12. The nurse is caring for a client who has been diaphoretic for the past 4 hours. The nurse plans to

A. offer the client the bedpan q 2 hours.
B. keep the emesis basin near the bedside.
*C. change the bed linens frequently.
D. offer oral care q 4 hours.

Reference: p. 919

Descriptors: 1. 37   2. 06   3. Application
            4. 4 = Planning   5. Moderate

13. A 78-year-old client who is weak on the third postoperative day requests that he be allowed to take a shower. Before the client takes a shower, the nurse should

A. place a non-skid mat on the shower floor.
B. stay near the room while the client showers.
C. be certain there is a lock on the shower room door.
*D. place a commode chair with the pan removed in the shower.

Reference: p. 920

Descriptors: 1. 37   2. 06   3. Application
            4. 5 = Implementation 5. Moderate

14. An adult client is to have a complete bed bath. Before beginning the bath, the nurse should

*A. offer the client the bedpan.
B. lower the client's bed to the lowest position.
C. assist the client to brush her teeth.
D. remove the client's hospital gown.

Reference: p. 921

Descriptors: 1. 37   2. 08   3. Application
            4. 5 = Implementation 5. Moderate

15. The nurse is bathing a client with an intravenous solution connected to the client's right forearm. The nurse should

A. disconnect the intravenous tubing to change the gown.
B. place the clean gown on the affected arm first.
*C. check the intravenous drip rate after the gown is changed.
D. remove both arms of the gown at the same time.

Reference: p. 926

Descriptors: 1. 37   2. 08   3. Application
            4. 5 = Implementation 5. Moderate

16. The nurse is preparing to give a "bag bath" to a 70-year-old hospitalized client. The nurse plans to

   A. towel dry the skin briefly after cleansing.
   *B. microwave the bag containing moistened washcloths.
   C. check the client's skin for irritation after the bath.
   D. use the towel in the bag to cleanse the entire body.

   Reference: p. 927

   Descriptors: 1. 37   2. 08   3. Application
   4. 4 = Planning   5. Moderate

17. A physician has ordered antiembolic stockings for an adult client. The client is sitting in a chair in the room when the nurse prepares to apply the stockings. The nurse plans to *first*

   A. measure the client's legs to ensure proper fit.
   B. ask the client to assist the nurse in the application of the stockings.
   C. massage the legs in brief, short strokes after the stockings are in place.
   *D. ask the client to lie in bed with legs elevated for 15 minutes before application.

   Reference: p. 927

   Descriptors: 1. 37   2. 09   3. Application
   4. 4 = Planning   5. Moderate

18. After removing a client's antiembolic stockings, the nurse observes a positive Homan's sign in the client's left leg. The nurse plans to

   A. document this finding in the client's record.
   B. massage the area with long smooth strokes.
   C. check the client's right leg for a positive Homan's sign.
   *D. contact the client's physician immediately.

   Reference: p. 929

   Descriptors: 1. 37   2. 04   3. Application
   4. 5 = Implementation 5. Moderate

19. The nurse is preparing to provide evening care to a client who has been on bedrest. An appropriate statement for the nurse to make before beginning the care is

   A. "Would you care for a backrub?"
   B. "Can you sit up for a backrub?"
   *C. "Now it is time for your backrub."
   D. "If you would like, I'll give you your backrub."

   Reference: p. 930

   Descriptors: 1. 37   2. 07   3. Application
   4. 5 = Implementation 5. Moderate

20. After completing the client's HS care, the nurse plans to

   A. ask the client if he needs a sleeping medication.
   B. elevate the bed to the highest position.
   C. keep the client's chair near the side of the bed.
   *D. be certain that the nurse's call light is within reach.

   Reference: pp. 930, 939

   Descriptors: 1. 37   2. 08   3. Application
   4. 4 = Planning   5. Moderate

21. The nurse is preparing to make an occupied bed for a client who is receiving oxygen for dyspnea. The nurse plans to

   A. discontinue the oxygen temporarily while making the bed.
   *B. keep the head of the bed elevated during the procedure.
   C. hold the dirty linens close to the body while discarding them into the laundry bag.
   D. adjust the client's bed to the lowest position before beginning.

   Reference: pp. 936, 938

   Descriptors: 1. 37   2. 08   3. Application
   4. 4 = Planning   5. Moderate

22. At 3 AM a hospitalized client complains of severe itching of his forearms and abdomen. The nurse caring for this client should

   A. use a small flashlight to observe the site of itching.
   B. turn on the bathroom light to observe the site of itching.
   C. open the drapes for available light and observe the site of itching.
   *D. turn on the bright lights above the bed long enough to observe the site of itching.

   Reference: p. 939

   Descriptors: 1. 37   2. 08   3. Application
   4. 5 = Implementation 5. Moderate

23. A 79-year-old thin client with arthritis has been admitted to the hospital following an automobile accident. To aid the client's comfort in bed the nurse plans to

   *A. provide the client with a sheepskin.
   B. use a rubberized mattress.
   C. cover the bottom sheet with a drawsheet.
   D. place a down comforter on top of the sheet.

   Reference: p. 940

   Descriptors: 1. 37   2. 10   3. Application
   4. 4 = Planning   5. Moderate

24. The nurse has instructed a 67-year-old client how to care for her dry skin. The nurse determines that the client needs *further* instructions when the client says,

    A. "Bubble baths can be very soothing."
    B. "I should bathe with soap less often."
  *C. "Wool clothing provides the least skin irritation."
    D. "I should try to increase my fluid intake."

Reference: pp. 940–941

Descriptors: 1. 37   2. 09   3. Application
            4. 6 = Evaluation   5. Moderate

25. An adolescent client has been instructed how to care for her skin which is prone to acne. The nurse determines that the client has understood the instructions when the client says

  *A. "I shouldn't squeeze or pick at the infected area."
    B. "I can use an emollient on my face over the area."
    C. "I can use an ultraviolet lamp daily to control the acne."
    D. "Wearing makeup doesn't affect the infected area."

Reference: p. 941

Descriptors: 1. 37   2. 09   3. Application
            4. 6 = Evaluation   5. Moderate

26. An adolescent client has received treatment for her acne which has resulted in erythema and some peeling of her skin. The nurse should advise the client to

    A. refrain from washing her skin more than twice daily.
    B. use an ultraviolet lamp once a day to aid the healing.
  *C. avoid sun exposure as sunburn could result.
    D. use heavy makeup to hide the skin tissues.

Reference: p. 941

Descriptors: 1. 37   2. 10   3. Application
            4. 5 = Implementation 5. Moderate

27. An adult client visits the clinic and complains of an itchy rash which developed after working in the yard. After providing the client with instructions about care of the rash, the nurse determines that the client understands the instructions when the client says,

    A. "Cool or cold baths can help alleviate the itching."
    B. "After washing the area, I should leave the soap on for a few minutes."
    C. "Medicated powders will help dry the area and stop the itching."
  *D. "Caladryl lotion may provide some relief."

Reference: p. 942

Descriptors: 1. 37   2. 10   3. Application
            4. 6 = Evaluation   5. Moderate

28. The nurse has instructed an 8-year-old client about the need for good oral hygiene. Besides brushing and flossing the teeth, the nurse encourages the client to consume foods which are rich in

  *A. vitamin D.
    B. riboflavin.
    C. folic acid.
    D. vitamin B_{12}.

Reference: p. 942

Descriptors: 1. 37   2. 10   3. Application
            4. 5 = Implementation 5. Moderate

29. An adult client with poor hygiene has been admitted to the hospital following an automobile accident. The nurse collaborates with the client and a formulates a goal with the client to perform a complete bath with assistance while hospitalized. The nurse evaluates progress toward accomplishing this goal by

    A. bathing the client to be certain the goal is reached.
    B. instructing the client why cleanliness is important.
  *C. observing the client while he is performing morning care.
    D. asking the client if he has completed his morning care.

Reference: p. 942

Descriptors: 1. 37   2. 10   3. Application
            4. 6 = Evaluation   5. Moderate

30. An adult client hospitalized with COPD is receiving continuous oxygen by nasal cannula. In preparing to assist the client with the morning care and range-of-motion exercises, a priority assessment for the nurse is to determine if the client

    A. can turn from side to side by herself.
  *B. needs frequent rest periods during the routine.
    C. exhibits disruptive behaviors during the bath.
    D. desires a backrub following the bath.

Reference: p. 943

Descriptors: 1. 37   2. 08   3. Application
            4. 2 = Assessment   5. Moderate

31. While working in a homeless shelter, an adult client with poor oral hygiene tells the nurse that he has severe bleeding gums and loose teeth. The nurse determines that the client is most likely experiencing

    A. dental caries.
    B. halitosis.
    C. gingivitis.
  *D. pyorrhea.

Reference: pp. 943–944

Descriptors: 1. 37   2. 10   3. Application
            4. 3 = Analysis/Diag.   5. Moderate

32. A thin adult client who has difficulty eating due to the side effects of chemotherapy has developed an inflammation of the oral mucosa. The nurse should explain to the client that this is a result of

A. vitamin B complex deficiencies.
B. anticholinergic drugs.
C. decreased fluid intake.
*D. chemotherapy medications.

Reference: p. 944

Descriptors: 1. 37   2. 10   3. Application
            4. 5 = Implementation 5. Moderate

33. The nurse is planning to provide oral care to an unconsious client in the critical care unit. To perform oral care, the nurse plans to use

A. a regular toothbrush and toothpaste.
B. soft cloths moistened with mouthwash.
*C. swabs moistened with normal saline.
D. a small toothbrush moistened with hydrogen peroxide.

Reference: pp. 944–945

Descriptors: 1. 37   2. 10   3. Application
            4. 4 = Planning   5. Moderate

34. The nurse is preparing to clean the dentures of an immobile homebound client. The nurse plans to

A. wear sterile gloves.
B. use hot water.
C. clean the dentures in the sink.
*D. rinse well after cleaning.

Reference: p. 945

Descriptors: 1. 37   2. 10   3. Application
            4. 4 = Planning   5. Moderate

35. A client is seen at home by the visiting nurse when the client tells the nurse that she hasn't any special denture soak in which to soak her dentures overnight. The nurse should instruct the client to use a solution of water and

A. baking soda.
B. bleach.
C. powdered toothpaste.
*D. vinegar.

Reference: p. 945

Descriptors: 1. 37   2. 10   3. Application
            4. 5 = Implementation 5. Moderate

36. The nurse has instructed a client how to floss his teeth for good oral hygiene. The nurse determines that the client needs *further* instructions when the client says,

A. "I should move the floss in an up and down motion."
B. "It's important that I rinse well after flossing."
*C. "If I have to, I should force the floss into the gum."
D. "I should keep about 1 to 1 1/2 inches of floss taut."

Reference: p. 945

Descriptors: 1. 37   2. 08   3. Application
            4. 6 = Evaluation   5. Moderate

37. The nurse plans to provide oral care to a dependent client. To remove the water from the client's oral cavity, the nurse plans to use a

A. bulb syringe.
*B. suction apparatus.
C. 10 mL. syringe.
D. dry washcloth.

Reference: p. 949

Descriptors: 1. 37   2. 10   3. Application
            4. 4 = Planning   5. Moderate

38. A 78-year-old client is scheduled for outpatient surgery to correct bilateral cataracts. The client tells the nurse that she is scared but that her daughter is with her. A priority nursing diagnosis for the client is

A. anticipatory grieving related to surgery.
B. risk for injury related to visual impairment.
C. sensory alteration due to stress.
*D. fear related to possible loss of vision.

Reference: p. 951

Descriptors: 1. 37   2. 10   3. Application
            4. 3 = Analysis/Diag.   5. Moderate

39. The nurse is assisting a weakened client with morning care. To cleanse the client's eyes the nurse should

A. use petroleum jelly around the edges of the eyes for moisture.
B. clean from the outer canthus to the inner canthus of the eyes.
*C. clean from the inner canthus to the outer canthus of the eyes.
D. use cool wet cotton balls to cleanse crustations.

Reference: p. 952

Descriptors: 1. 37   2. 08   3. Application
            4. 5 = Implementation 5. Moderate

40. The nurse is caring for a comatose client in a rehabilitation center. To care for the client's eyes, the nurse plans to

   *A. use artificial tear solution in the eyes q. 4 hours.
   B. place wet washcloths over the eyes to keep them moist.
   C. keep moistened cotton balls near the bedside to moisten the eyes.
   D. instill normal saline drops into the eyes at least once every 8 hours.

   Reference: pp. 952, 953

   Descriptors: 1. 37   2. 08   3. Application
                   4. 4 = Planning   5. Moderate

41. An alert adult client tells the nurse that the "dry air in the hospital" has made his nose stuffy. The nurse should

   A. use a bulb syringe to suction the client's nose.
   B. introduce a moistened cotton tip applicator into the client's nose.
   C. irrigate both nares with normal saline solution.
   *D. ask the client to blow gently into a soft tissue.

   Reference: pp. 952, 954

   Descriptors: 1. 37   2. 08   3. Application
                   4. 5 = Implementation 5. Moderate

42. The nurse prepares to clean a client's prescription eyeglasses. The nurse plans to dry the lenses with a

   A. sheet of toilet tissue.
   *B. soft cloth.
   C. sheet of paper towel.
   D. dry washcloth.

   Reference: p. 953

   Descriptors: 1. 37   2. 08   3. Application
                   4. 4 = Planning   5. Moderate

43. The nurse is caring for a client in the outpatient clinic who is wearing extended-wear contact lenses. The nurse should instruct the client that these type of lenses should be

   A. removed at least every other day.
   B. removed before sleeping.
   *C. cleansed at least once per week.
   D. replaced daily to prevent infection.

   Reference: p. 953

   Descriptors: 1. 37   2. 08   3. Application
                   4. 5 = Implementation 5. Moderate

44. An adult client is seen in the emergency room following an automobile accident. The client is wearing hard contact lenses and has suffered head and facial injuries. The nurse plans to

   A. remove the lenses with gentle suctioning.
   B. use gentle pressure to center the lens on the cornea.
   C. grasp the lens near the lower edge of the eye.
   *D. leave the lenses in place as injury may be present.

   Reference: pp. 953–954

   Descriptors: 1. 37   2. 08   3. Application
                   4. 4 = Planning   5. Moderate

45. The camp nurse has explained to a child why he must be inspected for ticks after spending the afternoon in the camp's wooded area. The nurse determines that the child understands the instructions when the child says that ticks can result in

   *A. Lyme disease.
   B. pediculosis.
   C. buleremia.
   D. fungal disease.

   Reference: p. 956

   Descriptors: 1. 37   2. 04   3. Application
                   4. 6 = Evaluation   5. Moderate

46. An African-American adolescent client asks the nurse how to care for her long hair which has been braided into small braids. The nurse should instruct the client that

   A. combs should be washed once a week.
   B. braids should be undone at least every other day.
   C. lubricants or oils should not be used on the braids.
   *D. hair should be washed as often as necessary.

   Reference: p. 956

   Descriptors: 1. 37   2. 09   3. Application
                   4. 5 = Implementation 5. Moderate

47. To assist an adult male client with a facial shave using a razor, the nurse should

   A. use firm, long strokes with gentle pressure.
   *B. wear gloves since contact with blood is possible.
   C. shave in the opposite direction of hair growth.
   D. rinse the face with an alcohol solution before beginning.

   Reference: p. 958

   Descriptors: 1. 37   2. 08   3. Application
                   4. 5 = Implementation 5. Moderate

48. The nurse has instructed an adult client with diabetes about proper foot care. The nurse determines that the client understood the instructions when the nurse observes the client

    A. cutting the toenails at the corners.
    B. trimming the toenails with scissors.
  *C. using a file to trim the toenails.
    D. walking barefoot in the hospital room.

Reference: p. 960

Descriptors: 1. 37   2. 08   3. Application
                4. 6 = Evaluation   5. Moderate

49. A sexually active female client asks the nurse about douching. The nurse instructs the client that vaginal douches should be used

    A. after every sexual contact.
    B. prior to a vaginal examination.
    C. with a vaginal deodorant.
  *D. no more than twice per week.

Reference: p. 964

Descriptors: 1. 37   2. 10   3. Application
                4. 5 = Implementation 5. Moderate

50. The nurse is preparing to administer a vaginal douche to a bedridden client. The nurse plans to

    A. use a bulb syringe for injection of the solution.
    B. raise the level of the bag during administration of the solution.
  *C. fill the douche bag with 1 to 2 quarts of solution.
    D. hold the douche bag about 12 inches above the hips.

Reference: p. 964

Descriptors: 1. 37   2. 10   3. Application
                4. 4 = Planning   5. Moderate

CHAPTER 38
Skin Integrity

1. The costs of treating clients with pressure ulcers are staggering. Some research has suggested that in nursing homes the proportion of clients with pressure ulcers is as great as

    A. 5%.
    B. 12%.
  *C. 23%.
    D. 48%.

Reference: p. 973

Descriptors: 1. 38   2. 02   3. Application
                4. 1 = No Process   5. Easy

2. While assessing a bedridden client at home for the presence of pressure ulcers, the nurse plans to inspect the client's

    A. buttocks.
    B. forearm.
    C. thigh.
  *D. coccyx.

Reference: p. 973

Descriptors: 1. 38   2. 03   3. Application
                4. 2 = Assessment   5. Moderate

3. While assessing a client in bed at home, the nurse inspects the client's environment for potential sources of friction which may lead to skin abrasions. The nurse should inspect the client's

  *A. bed sheets.
    B. blankets.
    C. bedside chair.
    D. bath linens.

Reference: p. 974

Descriptors: 1. 38   2. 03   3. Application
                4. 6 = Evaluation   5. Moderate

4. The nurse has instructed a group of nursing assistants about prevention of pressure ulcers due to shearing forces. The nurse determines that one of the nursing assistants needs *further* instructions when he says that shearing forces can be decreased when clients are

    A. lifted when moved up in bed.
    B. assisted by a bed trapeze during movement.
    C. transferred to a stretcher using bed linens.
  *D. pulled when they need to be moved up in bed.

Reference: pp. 974, 985

Descriptors: 1. 38   2. 07   3. Application
                4. 6 = Evaluation   5. Moderate

5. While bathing a client at home, the nurse observes blanching of the skin over the client's coccyx. The nurse documents this observation as a pressure ulcer in Stage

  *A. I.
    B. II.
    C. III.
    D. IV.

Reference: p. 975

Descriptors: 1. 38   2. 04   3. Interpretive
                4. 3 = Analysis/Diag.   5. Moderate

6. After turning a bedridden client from her side to her back, the nurse observes the area over the trochanter appears reddened. The nurse should document this observation as

A. Stage I ulcer.
B. ischemia.
C. eschar.
*D. hyperemia.

Reference: p. 975

Descriptors: 1. 38   2. 04   3. Interpretive
4. 3 = Analysis/Diag.   5. Moderate

7. A 75-year-old disoriented client is admitted to the hospital for surgery. The nurse observes damage to the subcutaneous tissue around the client's coccyx. The nurse determines that this stage of a pressure ulcer is Stage

A. I.
B. II.
*C. III.
D. IV.

Reference: p. 975

Descriptors: 1. 38   2. 04   3. Interpretive
4. 3 = Analysis/Diag.   5. Moderate

8. The nurse makes a home visit to a 70-year-old client with limited mobility. The client's daughter has been caring for the client following a total hip replacement. The nurse instructs the daughter that she should encourage the client to consume foods that are high in

A. vitamin D.
B. carbohydrates.
C. riboflavin.
*D. protein.

Reference: p. 975

Descriptors: 1. 38   2. 07   3. Application
4. 5 = Implementation 5. Moderate.

9. The nurse has instructed a caregiver of a bedridden incontinent client about care of the client to prevent pressure ulcers. The nurse determines that the caregiver understands the instructions when the caregiver says

A. "Ammonia in the urine can increase the risk of ulcers."
B. "I should change the linens at least every day."
C. "I should try to get an order for a catheter."
*D. "Moisture associated with incontinence is a risk factor."

Reference: pp. 977, 980

Descriptors: 1. 38   2. 07   3. Application
4. 6 = Evaluation   5. Moderate

10. The nurse is caring for an incoherent client with a pressure ulcer and begins to change the client's dressing. When the client grimaces and starts to cry the nurse should

A. try to calm the client with soothing words.
*B. provide comfort and pain relief.
C. perform the dressing change as quickly as possible.
D. delay the dressing change until the client is asleep.

Reference: p. 978

Descriptors: 1. 38   2. 08   3. Application
4. 5 = Implementation 5. Moderate

11. The nurse is caring for a group of clients in a nursing home. The nurse plans to inspect the at-risk clients for skin breakdown at least every

A. 4 hours.
B. 8 hours.
C. 16 hours.
*D. 24 hours.

Reference: p. 979

Descriptors: 1. 38   2. 07   3. Application
4. 4 = Planning   5. Moderate

12. While inspecting a pressure ulcer of a 90-year-old client, the nurse observes new tissue growth around the area which is pinkish-red in color. The nurse documents the presence of

A. epithelialization.
B. necrotic tissue.
*C. granulation.
D. hyperemia.

Reference: p. 980

Descriptors: 1. 38   2. 01   3. Application
4. 3 = Analysis/Diag.   5. Moderate

13. The nurse determines that the client who is at risk for developing a pressure ulcer is the client who has a/an

*A. albumin level of 2.5 mg/dL.
B. lymphocyte level of 2400/ mm^3.
C. hematocrit of 36 mg/dL.
D. hemoglobin of 14 mg/dL.

Reference: p. 980

Descriptors: 1. 38   2. 03   3. Application
4. 3 = Analysis/Diag.   5. Moderate

14. The nurse is using the Norton scale to assess a newly admitted 78-year-old client. An important assessment for the nurse to make using the Norton scale is

A. sensory deprivation.
B. presence of moisture.
C. friction and shear forces.
*D. activity level.

Reference: p. 982

Descriptors: 1. 38   2. 05   3. Application
4. 2 = Assessment   5. Moderate

15. The nurse admits a 90-year-old client from the hospital to the rehabilitation center following knee replacement surgery. The nurse observes a Stage III pressure ulcer on the client's heel. The priority nursing diagnosis for this client is

A. impaired mobility related to postoperative complications.
*B. impaired tissue integrity related to prolonged bedrest.
C. pain related to Stage III pressure ulcer.
D. impaired skin integrity related to advanced age.

Reference: p. 982

Descriptors: 1. 38   2. 06   3. Application
    4. 3 = Analysis/Diag.   5. Moderate

16. The nurse is assessing an 85-year-old client using the Braden scale for predicting pressure sores. An important aspect for the nurse to assess while using the Braden scale is

A. client's knowledge level.
B. dependence on caregivers.
*C. friction and shear potential.
D. physical condition.

Reference: p. 982

Descriptors: 1. 38   2. 05   3. Application
    4. 2 = Assessment   5. Moderate

17. Using the Braden scale for assessing a client for potential pressure ulcers, the nurse observes that the client eats over half of most meals and has at least four servings of protein daily. The nurse determines that the client's nutritional state is

A. very poor.
B. probably inadequate.
*C. probably adequate.
D. excellent.

Reference: p. 983

Descriptors: 1. 38   2. 05   3. Application
    4. 3 = Analysis/Diag.   5. Moderate

18. The nurse visits a 76-year-old client who is bedridden at home following abdominal surgery. The nurse observes that the client has a donut-type device under her buttocks. The nurse should instruct the client's caregiver that donut-type devices

A. prevent shearing forces which lead to abrasions.
*B. cause increased venous pressure and shouldn't be used.
C. need to be readjusted every 3 to 4 hours.
D. should have a pillowcase over them to reduce moisture.

Reference: p. 985

Descriptors: 1. 38   2. 07   3. Application
    4. 5 = Implementation 5. Moderate

19. The nurse observes a nursing student who is caring for a 79-year-old immobile client in bed. The nurse determines that the student is positioning the client correctly when the nurse observes the student

A. place a ring cushion under the client's sacrum.
B. pull the client up in bed to change the sheets.
C. keep the head of the bed elevated for most of the day.
*D. place a pillow under both calves of the client.

Reference: p. 985

Descriptors: 1. 38   2. 05   3. Application
    4. 6 = Evaluation   5. Moderate

20. The nurse is preparing to cleanse a pressure ulcer of a 91-year-old client. To accomplish the procedure, the nurse plans to obtain

A. warm, wet washcloths.
*B. normal saline solution.
C. hydrogen peroxide.
D. povidine solution.

Reference: p. 985

Descriptors: 1. 38   2. 07   3. Application
    4. 5 = Implementation 5. Moderate

21. While cleaning a pressure ulcer of a 74-year-old client, the nurse observes a thick white exudate and necrotic tissue. The nurse should

A. perform a wet-to-dry dressing.
B. obtain an irrigating device for suction.
C. collect a specimen of the tissue for laboratory analysis.
*D. notify the client's physician as soon as possible.

Reference: p. 986

Descriptors: 1. 38   2. 05   3. Application
    4. 5 = Implementation 5. Moderate

22. The nurse has instructed a caregiver of a 77-year-old client how to perform dressing changes on the client's pressure ulcer. The nurse determines that the caregiver understands the instructions when the caregiver says,

A. "I should pack the gauze tightly into the wound."
B. "It's important that the skin be kept moist."
*C. "I should use a moisture barrier ointment on the skin."
D. "Wet-to-dry dressings are used for pressure ulcers."

Reference: pp. 986, 988

Descriptors: 1. 38   2. 09   3. Application
    4. 6 = Evaluation   5. Moderate

23. The nurse has instructed a caregiver of an 82-year-old client with limited mobility about prevention of pressure ulcers. The nurse determines that the caregiver needs *further* instructions when the caregiver says,

    *A. "I should use hot water when I help her with her bath."
    B. "If she is incontinent, I should use a mild cleansing agent."
    C. "A nutritional supplement should be given if her dietary intake is inadequate."
    D. "It's important that bony prominences shouldn't be massaged."

Reference: p. 986

Descriptors: 1. 38   2. 09   3. Application
              4. 6 = Evaluation   5. Moderate

24. A student nurse is caring for a hospitalized client who is on a static flotation mattress for prevention of pressure ulcers. The nurse plans to explain to the student that one of the disadvantages of this type of mattress is that this mattress has

    *A. high moisture retention.
    B. high costs per day of use.
    C. low pressure reduction.
    D. low shear forces.

Reference: p. 987

Descriptors: 1. 38   2. 09   3. Application
              4. 5 = Implementation 5. Moderate

25. During a return demonstration of the "no-touch" technique of dressing change, the nurse determines that a client's caregiver understands the procedure when the nurse observes the caregiver

    A. don sterile gloves before beginning.
    B. clean the wound from the outer edges to the middle.
    C. touch the front center of the sterile gauze.
    *D. use clean gloves to pour the normal saline into a basin.

Reference: p. 988

Descriptors: 1. 38   2. 09   3. Application
              4. 6 = Evaluation   5. Moderate

CHAPTER 39
Activity

1. The type of joint in which the oval head of one bone fits into a shallow cavity of another, such as the wrist, is termed

    A. ball-and-socket.
    B. gliding.
    *C. condyloid.
    D. saddle.

Reference: p. 1000

Descriptors: 1. 39   2. 01   3. Factual
              4. 1 = No Process   5. Easy

2. When the nurse assists a bedridden client to perform range-of-motion exercises with her shoulders, the nurse should explain to the client that this type of joint is termed

    A. condyloid.
    B. hinge.
    C. pivot.
    *D. ball-and-socket.

Reference: p. 1000

Descriptors: 1. 39   2. 01   3. Factual
              4. 5 = Implementation 5. Easy

3. To assist a 73-year-old client to perform adduction, the nurse plans to move the client's

    *A. outstretched arm to a position alongside the body.
    B. leg inward with toes pointing toward the midline.
    C. neck and head upward towards the ceiling.
    D. leg in a circular motion.

Reference: p. 1000

Descriptors: 1. 39   2. 01   3. Factual
              4. 4 = Planning   5. Moderate

4. While assessing a comatose client, the nurse observes that the client's foot is rotated inward at the ankle. The nurse documents this as

    A. eversion.
    *B. inversion.
    C. pronation.
    D. dorsiflexion.

Reference: p. 1000

Descriptors: 1. 39   2. 01   3. Application
              4. 2 = Assessment   5. Easy

5. A 16-year-old client visits the emergency room after an automobile accident in which he fractured his nose. The nurse determines that the client has sustained an injury to his

    A. ligament.
    B. joint.
    C. tendon.
    *D. cartilage.

Reference: p. 1000

Descriptors: 1. 39   2. 02   3. Factual
              4. 2 = Assessment   5. Easy

6. Maintenance of posture, heat production, and motion are functions performed by the

    A. central nervous system.
    B. neurons.
    *C. muscle contractions.
    D. extensor reflexes.

Reference: p. 1003

Descriptors: 1. 39   2. 02   3. Factual
              4. 1 = No Process   5. Easy

7. A family member of a hospitalized client who has been on prolonged bedrest asks the nurse why range-of-motion exercises are being performed on her 80-year-old mother. The nurse should explain that prolonged bedrest can result in

*A. decreased muscle tonus.
B. decreased body mechanics.
C. increased muscle spasms.
D. increased skeletal pain.

Reference: p. 1004

Descriptors: 1. 39   2. 02   3. Application
            4. 5 = Implementation 5. Moderate

8. The nurse is preparing to assist an adult client to move from the bed to a chair. To increase balance and stability, the nurse should

A. use minor muscle groups to their fullest advantage.
*B. increase the base of support and lower the center of gravity.
C. rock forward and help push the client to the chair.
D. alter the client's center of gravity by raising his arms.

Reference: pp. 1004–1005, 1006

Descriptors: 1. 39   2. 08   3. Application
            4. 5 = Implementation 5. Moderate

9. An 8-year-old client visits the clinic and is diagnosed with an ear infection. He tells the mother and the nurse that he feels "dizzy." The nurse should explain to the client and his mother that the ear infection has affected a postural reflex termed the

A. proprioceptor sense.
B. kinesthetic sense.
C. gravitational sense.
*D. labyrinthine sense.

Reference: p. 1005

Descriptors: 1. 39   2. 03   3. Application
            4. 5 = Implementation 5. Moderate

10. The nurse makes a home visit to an 80-year-old postoperative client who is being cared for by his daughter. After instructing the caregiver about proper body mechanics, the nurse determines that the caregiver understands the instructions when the nurse observes the caregiver

*A. place her feet apart and flex at the knees when bending down.
B. bend over at the waist while keeping her knees straight.
C. reach out far in front of her to move the client to the bed.
D. lift the client from the chair to the bend while bending over.

Reference: pp. 1005–1006

Descriptors: 1. 39   2. 08   3. Application
            4. 6 = Evaluation   5. Moderate

11. The nurse visits a client in the home who is recovering from a stroke which left her partially paralyzed on her right side. After observing the client move successfully from the bed to the chair the nurse should reinforce the client by

A. encouraging the client to use caution when ambulating.
*B. congratulating the client on moving successfully.
C. showing the client how to perform isometric exercises.
D. demonstrating to the client how to stand in an erect position.

Reference: p. 1006

Descriptors: 1. 39   2. 03   3. Application
            4. 5 = Implementation 5. Moderate

12. The nurse is caring for a client with a diagnosis of achondroplasia. The nurse should assess the client for symptoms of

*A. dwarfism.
B. brittle bones.
C. bone deformities.
D. fractures.

Reference: p. 1007

Descriptors: 1. 39   2. 03   3. Application
            4. 3 = Analysis/Diag. 5. Moderate

13. A client visits the emergency room after falling while playing tennis. The injury has resulted in a partial tear to the ligaments around the ankle, known as a

A. spur.
B. dislocation.
*C. sprain.
D. strain.

Reference: pp. 1007, 1010

Descriptors: 1. 39   2. 03   3. Application
            4. 3 = Analysis/Diag. 5. Moderate

14. The nurse is performing a developmental assessment on a 3-year-old child. The nurse determines that the child needs further assessment when the nurse observes that the child cannot

*A. work a simple puzzle.
B. hop on one foot.
C. climb stairs without a handrail.
D. use a jump rope.

Reference: pp. 1008–1009

Descriptors: 1. 39   2. 03   3. Application
            4. 3 = Analysis/Diag. 5. Moderate

15. The nurse assesses a 3-month-old infant and determines that the infant is developing at a normal level when the nurse observes the infant in a prone position

  A. creep on all fours without assistance.
  B. pull herself up in the crib.
  C. roll over adeptly.
  *D. raise her head from the floor.

  Reference: p. 1008

  Descriptors: 1. 39   2. 03   3. Application
            4. 3 = Analysis/Diag.   5. Moderate

16. The nurse is caring for an adult client with multiple fractures and traction which requires prolonged bedrest. A priority nursing diagnosis for the client is

  A. risk for injury related to orthostatic hypotension.
  B. hypovolemia related to multiple trauma injuries.
  *C. potential for altered tissue perfusion related to immobility.
  D. risk for social isolation related to prolonged bedrest.

  Reference: p. 1011

  Descriptors: 1. 39   2. 07   3. Application
            4. 3 = Analysis/Diag.   5. Moderate

17. The nurse is caring for an adult client diagnosed with HIV disease who has a poor appetite and has limited mobility because of the disease. A priority nursing diagnosis for the client is

  A. impaired gas exchange related to decreased exercise.
  *B. altered nutrition: less than body requirements related to disease state.
  C. risk for activity intolerance related to decreased endurance.
  D. fluid volume excess related to dependent edema.

  Reference: p. 1013

  Descriptors: 1. 39   2. 07   3. Application
            4. 3 = Analysis/Diag.   5. Moderate

18. A 75-year-old client tells the nurse that she has been constipated. After giving the client instructions about how to decrease the constipation, the nurse determines that the client needs *further* instructions when the client says,

  A. "I should eat more vegetables and whole grain products."
  B. "It is important that I drink plenty of fluids throughout the day."
  *C. "It is OK if I have to strain when I try to have a BM."
  D. "Having a bedside commode might be helpful."

  Reference: p. 1014

  Descriptors: 1. 39   2. 10   3. Application
            4. 6 = Evaluation   5. Moderate

19. An adult client visits the clinic and tells the nurse that he is undergoing a great deal of stress on his new job and doesn't have time to exercise. The nurse should instruct the client that

  A. when the stressors at work are decreased, he'll have more time to exercise.
  B. fatigue from stress can contribute to the need for more rest.
  *C. regular exercise can be energizing and decrease the effects of stress.
  D. a regular program of strenuous exercise can be started when the stressors are gone.

  Reference: p. 1016

  Descriptors: 1. 39   2. 10   3. Application
            4. 5 = Implementation 5. Moderate

20. A client tells the nurse that she has joined a local club and is able to swim three times a week. The nurse should instruct the client that swimming is an

  A. isometric exercise that can improve muscle mass.
  *B. isotonic exercise that can improve cardiovascular function.
  C. isokinetic exercise that can improve respiratory function.
  D. isometric exercise that strengthens the quadriceps muscles.

  Reference: p. 1016

  Descriptors: 1. 39   2. 04   3. Application
            4. 5 = Implementation 5. Moderate

21. An adolescent client asks the nurse about exercises to increase his muscle mass and endurance. An appropriate exercise program for the nurse to suggest to the client is

  A. aerobics.
  B. stretching.
  C. isotonic.
  *D. strength.

  Reference: p. 1017

  Descriptors: 1. 39   2. 05   3. Application
            4. 5 = Implementation 5. Easy

22. A 65-year-old client who has been on bedrest for nine days asks the nurse why she needs to exercise when she doesn't feel like doing so. The nurse explains to the client about the reasons for the exercises and determines that the client understands the instructions when the client says that prolonged bedrest can lead to

  *A. increased cardiac workload.
  B. decreased heart rate.
  C. increased blood pressure.
  D. decreased cardiac stroke volume.

  References: p. 1017

  Descriptors: 1. 39   2. 05   3. Application
            4. 6 = Evaluation   5. Moderate

23. A 76-year-old client has been on bedrest for three days following abdominal surgery. The client has been receiving morphine. The nurse caring for this client plans to assess the client for

  A. contractures.
  B. ankylosis.
  *C. pneumonia.
  D. atrophy.

  Reference: p. 1019

  Descriptors: 1. 39   2. 05   3. Application
                4. 4 = Planning   5. Moderate

24. After several days of prolonged bedrest, the nurse ambulates the client for the first time from the bed to the chair. The client tells the nurse he is surprised how weak his legs have become. The nurse should explain to the client that prolonged bedrest can result in

  A. contractures.
  B. ankylosis.
  C. osteoporosis.
  *D. atrophy.

  Reference: p. 1019

  Descriptors: 1. 39   2. 05   3. Application
                4. 5 = Implementation 5. Moderate

25. After a period of prolonged bedrest, the physician tells the client that she has developed brittle bones. The nurse should explain to the client that the prolonged bedrest has resulted in

  *A. osteoporosis.
  B. contractures.
  C. fractures.
  D. atrophy.

  Reference: p. 1019

  Descriptors: 1. 39   2. 05   3. Application
                4. 5 = Implementation 5. Moderate

26. The nurse is planning to discuss osteoporosis with a group of perimenopausal women. Which of the following substances would be important for the nurse to include in the teaching plan to prevent or delay osteoporosis?

  A. Vitamin B-12
  *B. Calcium
  C. Beta-carotene
  D. Vitamin C

  Reference: p. 1020

  Descriptors: 1. 39   2. 05   3. Application
                4. 4 = Planning   5. Moderate

27. While caring for a client on prolonged bedrest, the nurse can help prevent the formation of renal calculi by

  A. decreasing the client's calcium intake.
  B. improving urinary alkalinity.
  *C. monitoring intake and output.
  D. encouraging Kegel's exercises.

  Reference: p. 1021

  Descriptors: 1. 39   2. 10   3. Application
                4. 4 = Planning   5. Easy

28. The nurse makes a home visit to a 70-year-old client who lives alone in a rural area. The client has limited mobility and limited financial resources and has recently been widowed after 40 years of marriage. A priority nursing diagnosis for the client is

  A. ineffective individual coping related to limited finances.
  B. powerlessness related to inability to perform self care activities.
  C. risk for infection related to limited mobility.
  *D. social isolation related to immobility.

  Reference: p. 1022

  Descriptors: 1. 39   2. 07   3. Application
                4. 3 = Analysis/Diag.   5. Moderate

29. A 40-year-old sedentary client who is overweight asks the nurse if he should begin a jogging program. The nurse should instruct the client that before beginning an exercise program, he should

  *A. have a preexercise medical examination.
  B. lose 10 pounds.
  C. have his cholesterol levels evaluated.
  D. wear the appropriate footwear to avoid injury.

  Reference: p. 1023

  Descriptors: 1. 39   2. 09   3. Application
                4. 5 = Implementation 5. Moderate

30. After several weeks of jogging, a client visits the clinic and complains of foot pain. The physician diagnoses the client with a torn tendon. The nurse should instruct the client to

  A. apply heat to the injured area.
  B. continue with his jogging routine.
  C. keep the foot in a dependent position.
  *D. apply a compression bandage to the foot.

  References: p. 1023

  Descriptors: 1. 39   2. 10   3. Application
                4. 5 = Implementation 5. Moderate

31. The nurse who wishes to serve as a role model for others and keep physically fit while preventing back injuries should

    A. lift a bedridden client when the nurse is fatigued.
    B. perform work activities even though shortness of breath occurs.
  *C. perform exercises for 30 minutes three times per week.
    D. keep weight to below normal for height.

References: p. 1023

Descriptors: 1. 39   2. 05   3. Application
               4. 5 = Implementation 5. Moderate

32. A 10-year-old client with cerebral palsy visits the clinic. The nurse observes the client sitting quietly but as the child reaches for a sucker on the counter, the client's hand begins to shake. The nurse determines that the client has

  *A. intentional tremors.
    B. postural tremors.
    C. athetosis.
    D. dystonia.

Reference: p. 1024

Descriptors: 1. 39   2. 06   3. Application
               4. 3 = Analysis/Diag. 5. Moderate

33. The nurse assesses a 65-year-old client and observes that the client is demonstrating brief, rapid, and jerky unpredictable movements. The nurse determines that the client is experiencing

    A. crepitation.
    B. dystonia.
    C. fasciculations.
  *D. chorea.

Reference: p. 1024

Descriptors: 1. 39   2. 06   3. Application
               4. 3 = Analysis/Diag. 5. Moderate

34. The nurse is caring for an adult client who demonstrates a grotesque and twisted posture while sitting in a chair. The nurse determines that the client is exhibiting symptoms of

    A. chorea.
  *B. dystonia.
    C. myoclonus.
    D. athetosis.

Reference: p. 1025

Descriptors: 1. 39   2. 06   3. Application
               4. 3 = Analysis/Diag. 5. Moderate

35. While assisting a 75-year-old client with range-of-motion exercises, the nurse hears a crunching sound while abducting the client's leg. The nurse documents this finding as

    A. subluxation.
    B. asymmetry.
  *C. crepitation.
    D. athetosis.

Reference: p. 1027

Descriptors: 1. 39   2. 06   3. Application
               4. 3 = Analysis/Diag. 5. Moderate

36. A client with cancer tells the nurse that he has decreased muscle mass in both legs. The nurse verifies the finding by measuring both legs and documents this finding as muscle

    A. flaccidity.
    B. hypertrophy.
    C. hemaplegia.
  *D. atrophy.

Reference: pp. 1027, 1029

Descriptors: 1. 39   2. 06   3. Application
               4. 3 = Analysis/Diag. 5. Moderate

37. The nurse is preparing to examine an adult client with hemiparesis following a stroke. The nurse anticipates that the client will have

  *A. weakness over one half of the body.
    B. paralysis over one half of the body.
    C. paralysis of both legs.
    D. spasticity of both arms.

Reference: p. 1029

Descriptors: 1. 39   2. 06   3. Application
               4. 3 = Analysis/Diag. 5. Moderate

38. The nurse is caring for an adult client on the third postoperative day and assesses the client's endurance by observing the client

    A. push the foot against the chair.
    B. pull himself up in bed.
  *C. turn himself in bed.
    D. push the nurse's palms apart.

Reference: p. 1029

Descriptors: 1. 39   2. 06   3. Application
               4. 2 = Assessment   5. Moderate

39. A 63-year-old client with advanced osteoarthritis and limited mobility tells the nurse that she feels badly because she "cannot even cook a simple meal" for her family because of her immobility. A priority nursing diagnosis is

   A. ineffective family coping related to the need for assistance.
   *B. self-esteem disturbance related to inability to meet role expectations.
   C. knowledge deficit related to appropriate exercise programs.
   D. risk for injury related to falls secondary to immobility.

   Reference: p. 1030

   Descriptors: 1. 39   2. 07   3. Application
                       4. 3 = Analysis/Diag.   5. Moderate

40. After his annual physical examination, the physician encourages an adult client to start a regular exercise program. The nurse plans goals with the client and an appropriate goal for this client is set: by the next visit, the client will

   A. document the need for an exercise program.
   B. maintain full joint range of motion.
   C. be exercising daily for 30 minutes.
   *D. list support systems to reinforce exercise efforts.

   Reference: p. 1031

   Descriptors: 1. 39   2. 10   3. Application
                       4. 4 = Planning   5. Moderate

41. The physician has ordered the bed of an adult client to be in the high-Fowler's position. The nurse plans to elevate the head of the client's bed

   A. 15°.
   B. 30°.
   C. 45°.
   *D. 90°.

   Reference: p. 1034

   Descriptors: 1. 39   2. 10   3. Application
                       4. 4 = Planning   5. Moderate

42. While caring for a client who is bedridden in a semi-Fowler's position, an important assessment for the nurse to make is assessment of the client's

   *A. sacrum.
   B. forearms.
   C. thighs.
   D. neck.

   Reference: p. 1034

   Descriptors: 1. 39   2. 06   3. Application
                       4. 2 = Assessment   5. Moderate

43. The nurse plans to turn a bedridden client to the Sim's position. The nurse should plan to

   A. place a pillow under the client's neck for support.
   *B. ensure that the two shoulders are in line with the hips.
   C. adduct the shoulder slightly in a flexed position.
   D. place a sandbag next to the client's ribcage.

   Reference: p. 1036

   Descriptors: 1. 39   2. 08   3. Application
                       4. 4 = Planning   5. Moderate

44. The nurse has instructed a nursing student how to perform passive range-of-motion exercises on an adult client. The nurse determines that the student needs *further* instructions when the student says,

   A. "It's important to cup my hand under the elbow to support it."
   B. "I should start gradually and work slowly."
   C. "If the client experiences pain, I should stop the exercises."
   *D. "The client's neck should be hyperextended towards the ceiling."

   Reference: p. 1037

   Descriptors: 1. 39   2. 10   3. Application
                       4. 6 = Evaluation   5. Moderate

45. The nurse is planning to move an obese client from a stretcher to the bed. Before transferring the client the nurse should plan to use a

   *A. transfer board.
   B. drawsheet.
   C. three carrier lift.
   D. trapeze.

   Reference: p. 1040

   Descriptors: 1. 39   2. 08   3. Application
                       4. 4 = Planning   5. Moderate

46. The nurse is preparing to transfer an adult client with left-sided weakness from the bed to a chair. The nurse should

   A. raise the bed to the highest level with head elevated.
   B. lower the head of the bed to the lowest position.
   C. stand behind the client while holding his waist.
   *D. position the chair facing the head or foot of the bed.

   Reference: pp. 1046–1047

   Descriptors: 1. 39   2. 08   3. Application
                       4. 5 = Implementation 5. Moderate

47. The nurse is caring for a client with limited mobility in her left leg and who uses a walker. The nurse determines that the client is using the walker correctly when the nurse observes the client

A. adjust the legs of the walker to a height of the client's diaphragm.
B. move the walker and the right leg forward 6 to 8 inches before the left leg.
*C. move the walker and the left leg forward 6 to 8 inches before the right leg.
D. use the walker for support when rising from a sitting to a standing position.

Reference: pp. 1053–1054

Descriptors: 1. 39   2. 08   3. Application
             4. 6 = Evaluation   5. Moderate

48. The nurse is planning to instruct a client how to walk with assistance of a cane. Which of the following should be included in the teaching plan? The client should

A. lean forward while walking with the cane.
B. hold the tip of the cane about 6 inches to the side of the foot.
C. start with a single-ended cane and move to a three-prong cane.
*D. hold the cane with elbows flexed on the unaffected side.

Reference: p. 1054

Descriptors: 1. 39   2. 10   3. Application
             4. 4 = Planning   5. Moderate

49. The nurse is caring for an adult client who will be using axillary crutches because of a fractured foot. The nurse should

*A. measure the distance of the client's axillary fold and add two inches.
B. instruct the client that support should come primarily from the axilla.
C. adjust the handgrips while the client keeps his elbows straight.
D. instruct the client to ambulate upstairs with the affected leg first.

Reference: pp. 1055–1056

Descriptors: 1. 39   2. 10   3. Application
             4. 5 = Implementation 5. Moderate

50. After a normal annual physical examination, a client tells the nurse she wishes to develop a personal exercise program. The nurse should *first*

A. identify support persons for the client.
*B. explore feasible exercise activities with the client.
C. discuss potential threats to the client's exercise program.
D. ask the client if she is really motivated to exercise.

Reference: p. 1058

Descriptors: 1. 39   2. 09   3. Application
             4. 5 = Implementation 5. Moderate

51. The nurse is caring for a client with rheumatoid arthritis and impaired physical mobility. An appropriate goal for the client is that the client will

A. identify four reasons why a daily exercise program is necessary.
B. demonstrate methods to conserve energy while exercising.
*C. perform activities of daily living with the greatest degree of independence possible.
D. maintain a pain-free status while exercising by using analgesic agents.

Reference: p. 1061

Descriptors: 1. 39   2. 10   3. Application
             4. 4 = Planning   5. Moderate

CHAPTER 40
Rest and Sleep

1. The nurse provides the postoperative client with an analgesic medication and darkens the room before the client goes to sleep for the night. The nurse's actions

A. help the client's circadian rhythm.
B. stimulate hormonal changes in the brain.
*C. decrease stimuli from the cerebral cortex.
D. alert the hypothalamus in the brain.

Reference: p. 1073

Descriptors: 1. 40   2. 02   3. Factual
             4. 5 = Implementation 5. Easy

2. Following an automobile accident which caused a head injury to an adult client, the nurse observes that the client sleeps for long periods of time. The nurse determines that the client has experienced injury to the

*A. hypothalamus.
B. thalamus.
C. cortex.
D. medulla.

Reference: p. 1073

Descriptors: 1. 40   2. 02   3. Application
             4. 3 = Analysis/Diag.   5. Moderate

3. A hospitalized adult client who routinely works from midnight until 8 AM has a temperature of 99.1°F at 4 AM The nurse determines that this is most likely due to

A. delta sleep.
B. slow brain waves.
C. pneumonia.
*D. circadian rhythm.

Reference: p. 1074

Descriptors: 1. 40   2. 02   3. Application
             4. 3 = Analysis/Diag.   5. Moderate

4. The nurse empties a Foley catheter bag for a client who appears to be asleep. The client is easily aroused when the nurse is close to the client's bedside. The nurse determines that the client was most likely in the non-REM sleep stage

A. I.
*B. II.
C. III.
D. IV.

Reference: pp. 1074–1075

Descriptors: 1. 40   2. 02   3. Application
          4. 3 = Analysis/Diag.   5. Moderate

5. An adult client visits the sleep disorder clinic for assessment. The nurse should instruct the client that routine studies for sleep disorders include an EEG and

*A. EOG.
B. KUB.
C. RUI..
D. CAT.

Reference: p. 1074

Descriptors: 1. 40   2. 02   3. Application
          4. 5 = Implementation 5. Moderate

6. A client who has just delivered a healthy newborn asks the nurse about newborn sleep patterns. The nurse should instruct the client that for the first three weeks newborns generally

A. have less REM sleep than older children.
B. demonstrate alert inactivity with eyes open.
*C. sleep 14 to 20 hours per day.
D. need two naps per day.

Reference: p. 1075

Descriptors: 1. 40   2. 04   3. Application
          4. 5 = Implementation 5. Moderate

7. When discussing newborn sleep patterns with a first-time mother, the client asks, "When will my baby sleep through the night?" The best response by the nurse is to instruct the client that newborns generally sleep through the night by

A. 1 month of age.
*B. 2–4 months of age.
C. 5–6 months of age.
D. 7–8 months of age.

Reference: p. 1077

Descriptors: 1. 40   2. 04   3. Application
          4. 5 = Implementation 5. Moderate

8. A client tells the nurse that she has been suffering from chronic fatigue even though she has been getting 10 to 12 hours of sleep each night. The nurse should assess the client for

A. dietary deficiencies.
B. lifestyle stressors.
*C. symptoms of illness.
D. parasomnia.

Reference: p. 1075

Descriptors: 1. 40   2. 04   3. Application
          4. 2 = Assessment   5. Moderate

9. A hospitalized adult client appears to be asleep when the nurse assesses the client's blood pressure. The nurse observes that the client's respirations are irregular and there is a 5 second period of apnea between respirations. The nurse determines that the client is experiencing

A. non-REM sleep.
*B. REM sleep.
C. narcolepsy.
D. sleep apnea.

Reference: p. 1075

Descriptors: 1. 40   2. 02   3. Application
          4. 3 = Analysis/Diag.   5. Moderate

10. The nurse is caring for a 3-year-old child hospitalized following an automobile injury. The nurse observes that the toddler awakens several times during the night. The nurse should

A. administer an ordered pain medication.
B. ask the child why he keeps awakening.
C. ask the child's mother to stay with her.
*D. provide comfort measures to the child.

Reference: p. 1077

Descriptors: 1. 40   2. 04   3. Application
          4. 5 = Implementation 5. Moderate

11. While discussing sleep patterns of school-age children with a group of parents, which of the following would be appropriate for the nurse to include in the teaching plan? School-age children

A. often have difficulty sleeping through the night.
B. may require less sleep during growth spurts.
*C. generally sleep 8 to 10 hours each night.
D. enjoy staying up late and sleeping late in the morning.

Reference: p. 1078

Descriptors: 1. 40   2. 04   3. Application
          4. 4 = Planning   5. Moderate

12. The nurse is planning a presentation for a group of adults age 65 or older about sleep. Which of the following should be included in the teaching plan?

   *A. Sleep–wakefulness patterns are often altered as one ages.
   B. The amount of REM sleep increases as one ages.
   C. Some adults have no Stage I sleep after the age of 60 years.
   D. Over the age of 60 years, clients are less likely to be disturbed by noise.

   Reference: p. 1079

   Descriptors: 1. 40   2. 04   3. Application
               4. 4 = Planning   5. Moderate

13. A client tells the nurse that he has been experiencing insomnia the past few days. The nurse should suggest to the client that an appropriate snack before bedtime to aid the sleep process is

   A. orange juice.
   *B. crackers.
   C. hot chocolate.
   D. bananas.

   Reference: p. 1080

   Descriptors: 1. 40   2. 03   3. Application
               4. 5 = Implementation 5. Moderate

14. An adult client has been diagnosed with hypothyroidism. The nurse should instruct the client that hypothyroidism can affect sleep by

   A. altering the brain waves.
   B. increasing the amount of REM sleep.
   C. causing chronic fatigue.
   *D. decreasing the amount of NREM sleep.

   Reference: p. 1080

   Descriptors: 1. 40   2. 03   3. Application
               4. 5 = Implementation 5. Moderate

15. A client diagnosed with asthma tells the nurse that he has frequent asthmatic attacks during sleep. The nurse should suggest to the client that he should try to

   A. eat a light protein snack before bedtime.
   B. take a one-hour nap during the day.
   *C. increase exercise to promote deep sleep.
   D. decrease the noise level in his environment.

   Reference: p. 1080

   Descriptors: 1. 40   2. 03   3. Application
               4. 5 = Implementation 5. Moderate

16. A client has been diagnosed with narcolepsy and given a prescription for an agrypnotic medication. The nurse should instruct the client that he should

   *A. take the medication faithfully each day.
   B. discontinue leisure activities for at least two weeks.
   C. reduce carbohydrate intake before bedtime.
   D. discontinue the medication when sleep patterns return to normal.

   Reference: pp. 1081, 1082

   Descriptors: 1. 40   2. 06   3. Application
               4. 5 = Implementation 5. Moderate

17. A 65-year-old client has suffered the loss of her husband of 40 years about two months ago. While visiting the client in her home, the client tells the nurse that she has been sleeping 14 to 16 hours per day and has no energy. The nurse determines that the client is most likely experiencing

   A. chronic illness.
   *B. hypersomnia.
   C. sleep apnea.
   D. narcolepsy.

   Reference: pp. 1081, 1082

   Descriptors: 1. 40   2. 03   3. Application
               4. 3 = Analysis/Diag.   5. Moderate

18. While caring for an adult male client, the nurse observes that the client is snoring while sleeping and stops breathing for 20 seconds between the snoring. The nurse determines that the client is most likely experiencing

   A. narcolepsy.
   B. hypersomnia.
   C. parasomnia.
   *D. sleep apnea.

   Reference: pp. 1081, 1082

   Descriptors: 1. 40   2. 05   3. Application
               4. 5 = Implementation 5. Moderate

19. A client tells the nurse that the physician has told her that her son suffers from bruxism. The nurse should explain to the client that the son

   A. talks while asleep.
   B. sleeps for long periods.
   *C. grinds the teeth while asleep.
   D. has nightmares.

   Reference: p. 1083

   Descriptors: 1. 40   2. 06   3. Application
               4. 5 = Implemenation 5. Moderate

20. A 65-year-old client complains to the nurse that she has no trouble falling asleep, but awakens every morning at 3 AM and cannot go back to sleep. The nurse determines that the client is most likely experiencing

   A. initial insomnia.
   *B. terminal insomnia.
   C. night terrors.
   D. sleep apnea.

   Reference: p. 1082

   Descriptors: 1. 40   2. 06   3. Application
                4. 3 = Analysis/Diag.   5. Moderate

21. The nurse is caring for a 45-year-old obese male client who is being treated for sleep apnea syndrome. The nurse instructs the client that sleep apnea syndrome is associated with

   *A. cardiac arrythmias.
   B. hypotension.
   C. chronic lung congestion.
   D. muscle tremors.

   References: p. 1082

   Descriptors: 1. 40   2. 06   3. Application
                4. 5 = Implementation 5. Moderate

22. A hospitalized client tells the nurse that he has been unable to sleep. To obtain more data related to the client's sleep problem, the nurse should first ask,

   A. "How many hours of sleep do you need?"
   B. "Do you take naps during the day?"
   *C. "Can you tell me about your sleep problem?"
   D. "Do you need a medication to help you sleep?"

   Reference: p. 1085

   Descriptors: 1. 40   2. 06   3. Application
                4. 2 = Assessment   5. Moderate

23. The nurse is caring for a 78-year-old client who lives with her daughter and tells the nurse she doesn't sleep much at night. The nurse should suggest to the client that to obtain more specific data on the client's sleep-wakefulness patterns, the client should

   *A. keep a sleep diary for 14 days.
   B. document what time she goes to sleep at night.
   C. ask her daughter to keep a graph of her sleep.
   D. record physical and mental activities before bedtime.

   Reference: pp. 1084, 1086

   Descriptors: 1. 40   2. 05   3. Application
                4. 5 = Implementation 5. Moderate

24. The nurse has instructed an adult client about how to keep a sleep diary. The nurse determines that the client understands the instructions when the client says,

   A. "I should keep records of the time I fall asleep."
   *B. "It's important to record my mental and physical activities."
   C. "It would be better if my husband kept the entire record for me."
   D. "It would be important to include any dreams I remember."

   Reference: p. 1086

   Descriptors: 1. 40   2. 06   3. Application
                4. 6 = Evaluation   5. Moderate

25. A 68-year-old client who has had chronic insomnia most of her adult life tells the nurse that sometimes she wakes up because her legs are jerking. The nurse determines that the client is most likely experiencing

   A. vitamin D deficiency.
   B. restless leg syndrome.
   C. nocturnal enuresis.
   *D. nocturnal myoclonus.

   Reference: p. 1086

   Descriptors: 1. 40   2. 04   3. Application
                4. 3 = Analysis/Diag.   5. Moderate

26. The nurse is caring for a client who experiences frequent somnambulism while sleeping in a second floor bedroom. A priority nursing diagnosis for this client is

   A. knowledge deficit related to ways to control the somnambulism.
   *B. risk for injury related to somnambulism and environment.
   C. anxiety related to fear of falling out of bed during the night.
   D. impaired social interaction related to fear of somnambulism.

   Reference: p. 1086

   Descriptors: 1. 40   2. 07   3. Application
                4. 3 = Analysis/Diag.   5. Moderate

27. A 39-year-old client is seen in the clinic because she has been sleeping 14 to 16 hours per day. The client states that she is "depressed because my mother died from cancer two months ago." A priority nursing diagnosis for this client is

   A. altered sleep patterns related to depression and grief response.
   B. depression related to loss of mother and excessive sleeping.
   C. sleep pattern disturbance related to inability to resolve grief.
   *D. sleep pattern disturbance related to grief process and loss of mother.

   Reference: p. 1087

   Descriptors: 1. 40   2. 07   3. Application
                4. 3 = Analysis/Diag.   5. Moderate

28. While making a home visit to a 76-year-old client, the client tells the nurse that she often has trouble sleeping and then is "tired all day." The nurse should instruct the client to

A. watch television in bed before going to sleep.
B. take a short nap if she feels fatigued.
*C. keep a routine of waking and sleeping.
D. eat a light protein snack before bedtime.

Reference: p. 1089

Descriptors: 1. 40   2. 06   3. Application
4. 5 = Implementation 5. Moderate

29. A first-time mother complains to the nurse that her 3-year-old refuses to go to bed at night and frequently gets out of bed for water and snacks during the evening. The nurse should instruct the client that the family should

A. avoid snacks before bedtime.
B. allow the child to stay up until sleepy.
C. decrease the temperature in the child's room.
*D. follow a bedtime ritual every evening.

Reference: p. 1089

Descriptors: 1. 40   2. 08   3. Application
4. 5 = Implementation 5. Moderate

30. To promote sleep for a hospitalized adult client, the nurse encourages the client to

A. drink a large glass of water 2 hours before bedtime.
B. exercise for 15 minutes before bedtime.
C. refrain from eating carbohydrates before bedtime.
*D. practice meditation before bedtime.

Reference: p. 1099

Descriptors: 1. 40   2. 08   3. Application
4. 5 = Implementation 5. Moderate

31. A hospitalized client tells the nurse that she finds that early morning napping makes her feel better during the day. The nurse should instruct the client that morning naps

A. may interfere with nighttime sleep.
*B. are often associated with REM sleep.
C. can help the client cope with hospitalization.
D. are usually a sign that the client is healing.

Reference: p. 1091

Descriptors: 1. 40   2. 08   3. Application
4. 5 = Implementation 5. Moderate

32. An adult client is given a prescription for a sedative-hypnotic to aid in sleep. Following instructions about the medication, the nurse determines that the client understands the instructions when he says,

A. "I can continue to take my Benadryl while on this medication."
B. "This medication has no effect on REM sleep stages."
*C. "I should only take this medication temporarily."
D. "If the medication loses its effect, I can increase the dosage later."

Reference: p. 1091

Descriptors: 1. 40   2. 09   3. Application
4. 6 = Evaluation   5. Moderate

33. The nurse is caring for an 84-year-old client who has been taking a hypnotic drug for several years. The client tells the nurse that she quit taking the medication yesterday as it was no longer effective. The nurse should assess the client for

A. nausea.
B. diarrhea.
*C. restlessness.
D. decreased pulse.

Reference: p. 1091

Descriptors: 1. 40   2. 04   3. Application
4. 2 = Assessment   5. Moderate

34. The nurse is caring for an adult client who is being discharged from the hospital with a prescription for a sedative-hypnotic drug. The nurse plans to instruct the client to

A. take the medication every evening whether it is needed or not.
B. drink a glass of milk while taking the medication.
*C. avoid alcoholic beverages while on the medication.
D. contact the physician if the drug is no longer effective.

Reference: p. 1091

Descriptors: 1. 40   2. 09   3. Application
4. 5 = Implementation 5. Moderate

35. The nurse is caring for a client who had a restless night due to postoperative pain. When the nurse enters the room at 7 AM for morning vital signs, the client is sound asleep. The nurse should

A. document that the client was asleep at 7 AM and leave the room.
B. assess the client's vital signs while trying not to disturb him.
C. ask the night shift nurse what the client's vital signs were at 4 AM.
*D. allow the client to rest and assess the vital signs later in the morning.

Reference: p. 1092

Descriptors: 1. 40   2. 08   3. Application
4. 5 = Implementation 5. Moderate

36. A client visits the clinic and tells the nurse that he has recently taken a new job and has had difficulty falling asleep for the past few days. The nurse determines that the client is most likely experiencing

   A. transitional insomnia.
   B. sleep deprivation.
   C. parasomnia.
  *D. transient insomnia.

Reference: p. 1093

Descriptors: 1. 40   2. 09   3. Application
           4. 3 = Analysis/Diag.   5. Moderate

37. A client who smokes one pack of cigarettes every day tells the nurse that he has had trouble falling asleep for the past few nights because he is worried about possible loss of his job. The nurse instructs the client to

  *A. decrease or stop smoking during the day.
   B. practice relaxation techniques during the day.
   C. exercise for 30 minutes before bedtime.
   D. try to fall asleep even if not sleepy.

Reference: p. 1094

Descriptors: 1. 40   2. 08   3. Application
           4. 5 = Implementation 5. Moderate

38. The nurse has received an adult client who has been transferred from an intensive care unit where his sleep was often interrupted. The nurse should assess the client for

   A. jitteriness.
   B. nausea.
   C. hallucinations.
  *D. irritability.

Reference: p. 1094

Descriptors: 1. 40   2. 09   3. Application
           4. 2 = Assessment   5. Moderate

39. A 79-year-old client tells the nurse that she has been taking Valium for several months but still feels tired after 8 hours of sleep. The nurse should assess the client for

   A. hallucinations.
  *B. depression.
   C. nightmares.
   D. twitching.

Reference: p. 1094

Descriptors: 1. 40   2. 06   3. Application
           4. 2 = Assessment   5. Moderate

40. The nurse is caring for a hospitalized client who needs frequent assessments during the night. The nurse should plan to

   A. leave the overhead light on throughout the night.
   B. make the assessments while using a penlight.
  *C. place a soft nightlight near the client's bedside.
   D. use a bright flashlight when assessments are performed.

Reference: p. 1095

Descriptors: 1. 40   2. 08   3. Application
           4. 4 = Planning   5. Moderate

CHAPTER 41
Comfort

1. A client has suffered from a paper cut while writing a letter. The nurse should explain to the client that this type of cut results in pain termed

   A. somatic.
   B. referred.
  *C. cutaneous.
   D. deep.

Reference: p. 1103

Descriptors: 1. 41   2. 01   3. Application
           4. 5 = Implementation 5. Moderate

2. Following abdominal surgery, an adult client requests pain medication for incisional pain. The nurse determines that the client is most likely experiencing pain termed

  *A. visceral.
   B. referred.
   C. somatic.
   D. endorphic.

Reference: p. 1104

Descriptors: 1. 41   2. 01   3. Application
           4. 3 = Analysis/Diag.   5. Moderate

3. An adult client visits the emergency room complaining of pain that radiates down his left arm. The nurse determines that the client is most likely experiencing pain termed

   A. psychogenic.
  *B. referred.
   C. transmitted.
   D. cutaneous.

Reference: p. 1104

Descriptors: 1. 41   2. 01   3. Application
           4. 3 = Analysis/Diag.   5. Moderate

4. An injury to human tissue causes the release of histamine and pain receptors are then stimulated by

   A. substance K.
   *B. bradykinin.
   C. endorphins.
   D. enkephalins.

   Reference: p. 1104

   Descriptors: 1. 41   2. 01   3. Factual
                4. 1 = No Process   5. Moderate

5. The nurse is caring for a client following an automobile accident in which the client's sciatic nerve was partially injured. The client complains of a burning pain around the palms of his hands. The nurse determines that the client is most likely experiencing

   *A. causalgia.
   B. neuralgia.
   C. myoclonus.
   D. arthritis.

   Reference: p. 1105

   Descriptors: 1. 41   2. 03   3. Application
                4. 3 = Analysis/Diag.   5. Moderate

6. A client is has been diagnosed with trigeminal neuralgia. An important assessment for the nurse to make is the client's

   A. dependence on medications.
   B. weight-bearing joints.
   *C. level of exhaustion.
   D. intervertebral discs.

   Reference: p. 1105

   Descriptors: 1. 41   2. 03   3. Interpretive
                4. 2 = Assessment   5. Moderate

7. Following an above-the-knee amputation as a result of diabetic complications, the client continues to complain of pain in his amputated leg. The nurse determines that the client is experiencing pain termed

   A. psychosomatic.
   B. referred.
   C. myofascial.
   *D. phantom limb.

   Reference: pp. 1105, 1106

   Descriptors: 1. 41   2. 03   3. Application
                4. 3 = Analysis/Diag.   5. Moderate

8. Using the gate control theory of pain, an important nursing measure for a client in pain is for the nurse to

   A. position the client with several pillows.
   B. assist the client with relaxation techniques.
   C. provide pain medications as ordered.
   *D. give the client a gentle backrub.

   Reference: p. 1107

   Descriptors: 1. 41   2. 04   3. Application
                4. 5 = Implementation 5. Moderate

9. The nurse plans to instruct an adult client about relaxation techniques to help relieve postoperative pain. Which of the following should be included in the teaching plan?

   A. Relaxation techniques can help close the pain gate.
   B. Meditation reduces the pain threshold.
   *C. Endorphins are released during relaxation.
   D. Exhaustion can be minimized with neuromuscular relaxation.

   Reference: p. 1108

   Descriptors: 1. 41   2. 07   3. Application
                4. 4 = Planning   5. Moderate

10. The nurse is caring for a client with terminal cancer and the client reports that no matter what she does, the pain is never relieved. The nurse determines that the client is experiencing pain termed

    *A. intractable.
    B. intolerable.
    C. diffuse.
    D. acute.

    Reference: p. 1109

    Descriptors: 1. 41   2. 03   3. Application
                 4. 3 = Analysis/Diag.   5. Moderate

11. The nurse is planning a presentation on the topic of pain to a group of nursing students caring for terminally ill clients. Which of the following should be included in the nurse's teaching plan?

    A. Infants have little perception of pain until they are older.
    B. Pain in older adults is viewed as a normal part of the aging process.
    *C. Individuals who have experienced more pain in their life have increased sensitivity.
    D. Rested and relaxed individuals may experience pain in an acute manner.

    Reference: pp. 1112–1113

    Descriptors: 1. 41   2. 04   3. Application
                 4. 1 = No Process   5. Moderate

12. The nurse has instructed a postoperative client about pain and pain relief methods. The nurse determines that the client needs *further* instructions when the client says,

    A. "If I am feeling pain, I should ask for my ordered pain medication."
    B. "All pain is real, regardless of its cause, and there is a physical and mental component."
    *C. "If I ask for something for pain, I may become addicted to the medication."
    D. "Lack of pain expression does not necessarily mean lack of pain."

    Reference: p. 1114

    Descriptors: 1. 41   2. 04   3. Application
                 4. 6 = Evaluation   5. Moderate

13. A family member tells the nurse that no matter what interventions are provided for a postoperative client, the client continues to complain of pain at the incision site. The best response by the nurse is to tell the family member,

   *A. "Individuals with prolonged pain have an increasingly low pain tolerance."
   B. "Lying about the pain, or malingering, is common among adults."
   C. "People in pain should be taught to have a higher pain tolerance."
   D. "Pain is usually the result of an emotional or psychologic problem."

   Reference: p. 1114

   Descriptors: 1. 41   2. 02   3. Application
                4. 5 = Implementation 5. Moderate

14. A postoperative client tells the nurse that he is having pain. To obtain more data, an appropriate response by the nurse is

   A. "Do you need your pain medication now?"
   *B. "Tell me more about your pain."
   C. "When did you last receive your pain medication?"
   D. "Tell me where the pain is located."

   Reference: p. 1115

   Descriptors: 1. 41   2. 05   3. Application
                4. 2 = Assessment   5. Moderate

15. The nurse is discussing pain control with a client who is scheduled for abdominal surgery. The nurse should include a discussion about the client's

   A. family members support.
   B. level of education.
   *C. expectations for pain relief.
   D. pain tolerance levels.

   Reference: p. 1115

   Descriptors: 1. 41   2. 05   3. Application
                4. 5 = Implementation 5. Moderate

16. The nurse is caring for a 4-year-old hospitalized child following cardiac surgery. To assess the child's pain level the nurse should

   A. assess the client's vital signs and other symptoms of pain.
   *B. ask the child to compare his pain to a series of faces ranging from a broad smile to a grimace.
   C. ask the family members what symptoms in the child indicate pain.
   D. ask the child's mother to record the pain in a pain diary.

   Reference: pp. 1115, 1120

   Descriptors: 1. 41   2. 05   3. Application
                4. 5 = Implementation 5. Moderate

17. The nurse has presented the topic of pain to a group of adults age 65 years and older. The nurse determines that one of the participants needs *further* instructions when he says,

   *A. "People over 65 years of age have decreased pain sensitivity and tolerance."
   B. "Boredom and loneliness can affect a person's perception of pain."
   C. "Having pain is not an expected outcome of the aging process."
   D. "The expression of pain varies based on a person's culture or ethnic background."

   Reference: p. 1119

   Descriptors: 1. 41   2. 05   3. Application
                4. 6 = Evaluation   5. Moderate

18. The nurse is caring for an adult client on the first postoperative day following thoracic surgery. The client is reluctant to ask for pain medication yet appears to be in obvious pain. The priority nursing diagnosis for this client is

   A. ineffective individual coping related to past pain experience.
   *B. pain: postoperative related to fear of taking prescribed analgesics.
   C. pain related to decreased blood supply to the thoracic cavity.
   D. knowledge deficit related to appropriate pain management techniques.

   Reference: p. 1120

   Descriptors: 1. 41   2. 06   3. Application
                4. 3 = Analysis/Diag.   5. Moderate

19. The nurse is caring for a hospitalized client who is quadriplegic and has had surgery on his right arm. The priority nursing diagnosis for this client is

   A. chronic pain related to quadraplegia and surgery.
   B. fear related to possible outcome of surgery.
   *C. risk for injury related to decreased pain sensation.
   D. anxiety related to heightened pain anticipation.

   Reference: p. 1120

   Descriptors: 1. 41   2. 06   3. Application
                4. 3 = Analysis/Diag.   5. Moderate

20. A client with terminal cancer tells the nurse she has a great deal of pain and the medication is not working. She asks the nurse, "Why is God punishing me like this?" A priority nursing diagnosis for the client is

A. acute pain related to ineffective analgesia.
B. impaired physical mobility related to acute pain episode.
C. risk of self-directed violence related to loss of will to live.
*D. spiritual distress related to belief that God is causing pain as punishment.

Reference: p. 1122

Descriptors: 1. 41   2. 06   3. Application
            4. 3 = Analysis/Diag.   5. Moderate

21. The nurse has instructed a family member about caring for her father, who is experiencing chronic pain from osteoarthritis. The nurse determines that the caregiver needs *further* instructions when the caregiver says,

*A. "I should leave him in a darkened room with as little stimuli as possible."
B. "It's important to prevent him from becoming constipated."
C. " I should encourage him to change positions frequently."
D. "It's important that he be kept well hydrated throughout the day."

Reference: p. 1122

Descriptors: 1. 41   2. 07   3. Application
            4. 6 = Evaluation   5. Moderate

22. The nurse is caring for a client in active labor who is using the Lamaze method to cope with the labor pain. The nurse determines that the client is using the method appropriately when the nurse observes the client using

A. imagery.
B. biofeedback.
C. shallow breathing.
*D. distractions.

Reference: p. 1124

Descriptors: 1. 41   2. 07   3. Application
            4. 6 = Evaluation   5. Moderate

23. The nurse is planning to instruct a client with chronic pain from arthritis about the use of imagery to decrease pain sensation. The nurse should *first*

A. ask the client to take a cleansing deep breath.
*B. identify the problem or goal.
C. encourage images of the desired state of well-being.
D. inform the client about external healing therapies.

Reference: p. 1124

Descriptors: 1. 41   2. 07   3. Application
            4. 5 = Implementation 5. Moderate

24. The nurse is planning a presentation about relaxation techniques to a group of young adults. Which of the following would be important for the nurse to include in the teaching plan?

A. Relaxation therapies do not provide distraction from pain.
B. Acute pain situations benefit more from relaxation therapies than chronic pain.
*C. Relaxation is most effective when combined with slow, deep breathing.
D. Massage during relaxation techniques improve the effectiveness.

Reference: p. 1125

Descriptors: 1. 41   2. 07   3. Application
            4. 4 = Planning   5. Moderate

25. To perform contralateral stimulation for a client with pain in his right leg, the nurse should provide

A. back massage.
B. heat to the affected area.
*C. skin stimulation to the left leg.
D. accupressure to the scalp area.

Reference: p. 1122

Descriptors: 1. 41   2. 07   3. Application
            4. 5 = Implementation 5. Moderate

26. The nurse is preparing to use therapeutic touch with a client experiencing postoperative pain. The nurse should *first*

A. obtain a physician's order for the treatment.
*B. center himself/herself.
C. visualize the energy field.
D. restore balance to the client.

Reference: p. 1127

Descriptors: 1. 41   2. 07   3. Application
            4. 5 = Implementation 5. Moderate

27. Which of the following is true about pain management practices among physicians and nurses?

A. Physicians frequently prescribe higher analgesic doses than necessary.
B. Nurses frequently overestimate the client's need for pain medication.
*C. Nurses frequently give low priority to a client's pain management.
D. Physicians frequently underestimate the duration of analgesics.

Reference: p. 1128

Descriptors: 1. 41   2. 09   3. Application
            4. 1 = No Process   5. Moderate

28. The nurse is planning to instruct a client about the use of nonsteroidal antiinflammatory analgesics for arthritis pain. Which of the following should be included in the teaching plan?

   A. Clients with bleeding disorders can take these medications safely.
   B. Respiratory depression is a common side effect of these medications.
   C. Constipation can result from overuse of these medications.
   *D. These medications can cause gastric irritation.

   Reference: p. 1128

   Descriptors: 1. 41   2. 05   3. Application
               4. 4 = Planning   5. Moderate

29. The nurse assesses a client 3 hours after receiving morphine for pain. The nurse determines that the client's sedation level is 3. The nurse should

   A. contact the physician for an order for naloxone.
   *B. withhold the next dose of medication until the client is less sedated.
   C. assess the client's respiratory rate for a full minute.
   D. stimulate the client and ask him to breathe deeply.

   Reference: p. 1129

   Descriptors: 1. 41   2. 08   3. Application
               4. 5 = Implementation 5. Moderate

30. A client with terminal cancer has been taking a prescribed opioid medication for pain relief for two months. The nurse should assess the client for

   *A. constipation.
   B. respiratory depression.
   C. addiction.
   D. hypertension.

   Reference: p. 1129

   Descriptors: 1. 41   2. 08   3. Application
               4. 2 = Assessment   5. Moderate

31. An Asian-American client appears in obvious pain following abdominal surgery; however, he rarely asks for pain medication. The nurse should instruct the client that for the analgesic to be the most effective, the client should

   A. ask for the medication only when the pain is severe.
   B. take the medication every 4 hours as ordered.
   *C. request pain medication before the pain gets severe.
   D. take the pain medication only if other measures are ineffective.

   Reference: p. 1130

   Descriptors: 1. 41   2. 05   3. Application
               4. 5 = Implementation 5. Moderate

32. A client has an intravenous patient-controlled analgesia pump (PCA) with morphine following thoracic surgery. The nurse should instruct the client that one of the primary advantages of patient-controlled analgesia is that

   A. the client can administer the medication whenever the client desires.
   B. a family member can help with administration of the medication.
   C. the nurse can more accurately assess the effectiveness of the analgesia.
   *D. consistent analgesic blood levels are maintained.

   Reference: p. 1133

   Descriptors: 1. 41   2. 10   3. Application
               4. 5 = Implementation 5. Moderate

33. A client is transferred from the operating room to the nursing unit following abdominal surgery. The client has a continuous epidural in place for analgesia. The nurse should assess the client for

   *A. urine retention.
   B. hallucinations.
   C. hypertension.
   D. tolerance.

   Reference: p. 1136

   Descriptors: 1. 41   2. 08   3. Application
               4. 2 = Assessment   5. Moderate

34. The physician has suggested to an adult client with intractable pain that a neurectomy can be used to treat the pain. The nurse determines that the client understands the procedure when the client says that this procedure

   A. is indicated for localized pain in the neck area.
   *B. may result in total loss of sensation and some paralysis.
   C. is useful for phantom limb pain.
   D. requires incision of the spinal cord.

   Reference: p. 1137

   Descriptors: 1. 41   2. 09   3. Application
               4. 6 = Evaluation   5. Moderate

35. A client with terminal cancer is being treated with continuous morphine epidural anesthesia. The nurse should tell the caregiver that an appropriate drug to have on hand in case of respiratory depression is

   A. Thorazine.
   B. Naproxen.
   C. Demerol.
   *D. Narcan.

   Reference: p. 1141

   Descriptors: 1. 41   2. 10   3. Application
               4. 5 = Implementation 5. Moderate

CHAPTER 42
Nutrition

1. A client is trying to reduce her weight by 6 pounds over three weeks. Her normal caloric intake is 1800 calories per day. The nurse should help the client plan a diet with a caloric intake of

   A. 1000 calories.
   B. 1100 calories.
   C. 1200 calories
   *D. 1300 calories.

   Reference: p. 1152

   Descriptors: 1. 42   2. 01   3. Application
   4. 4 = Planning   5. Moderate

2. A diabetic client with hypoglycemia needs an immediate source of sugar to raise his blood sugar level. The nurse should offer the client a

   A. polysaccharide.
   B. starch
   *C. monosaccharide.
   D. dissacharide.

   Reference: p. 1153

   Descriptors: 1. 42   2. 02   3. Application
   4. 5 = Implementation 5. Moderate

3. The hormones which are responsible for keeping serum glucose levels fairly constant during both feasting and fasting are insulin and

   A. adrenalin.
   *B. glucagon.
   C. thyroxin.
   D. aldosterone.

   Reference: p. 1153

   Descriptors: 1. 42   2. 01   3. Application
   4. 1 = No Process   5. Moderate

4. An adult client complains to the nurse that he experiences constipation. The nurse should suggest to the client that he consume extra

   A. milk products.
   B. eggs.
   *C. carrots.
   D. tomatoes.

   Reference: p. 1154

   Descriptors: 1. 42   2. 02   3. Application
   4. 5 = Implementation 5. Moderate

5. The nurse is caring for a newly diagnosed diabetic client. To help improve the client's glucose tolerance level, the nurse instructs the client to consume

   A. nuts.
   B. milk.
   C. fish.
   *D. oatmeal.

   Reference: p. 1154

   Descriptors: 1. 42   2. 02   3. Application
   4. 5 = Implementation 5. Moderate

6. The nurse is planning a presentation to a group of adult clients on the topic of healthy diets. Which of the following would be important for the nurse to include in the teaching plan?

   *A. Heart disease and obesity have been correlated with high-fat diets.
   B. Protein deficiency is common in the United States.
   C. Dietary experts recommend eating more animal protein and less vegetable protein.
   D. Carbohydrate intake should comprise 30% of the daily diet.

   Reference: p. 1154

   Descriptors: 1. 42   2. 02   3. Application
   4. 4 = Planning   5. Moderate

7. A client following a vegetarian diet asks the nurse what he can do to get more protein with a meal that consists of a corn tortilla and refried beans. The nurse should suggest complementary protein such as

   A. lettuce and tomato salad.
   B. cooked spinach.
   *C. lentil rice soup.
   D. granola bar.

   Reference: p. 1155

   Descriptors: 1. 42   2. 02   3. Application
   4. 5 = Implementation 5. Moderate

8. One month following major abdominal surgery, a 75-year-old client tells the nurse that she has lost 20 pounds. The nurse should assess the client for

   A. positive nitrogen balance.
   *B. negative nitrogen balance.
   C. anabolism.
   D. catabolism.

   Reference: p. 1155

   Descriptors: 1. 42   2. 02   3. Application
   4. 2 = Assessment   5. Moderate

9. The nurse is caring for a 4-year-old child who has had frequent infections during the last year. The nurse should instruct the client's mother that to help ward off infections, the mother should offer the child foods that are high in

   A. carbohydrate.
   B. fat.
   *C. protein.
   D. water soluble fiber.

   Reference: pp. 1155–1156

   Descriptors: 1. 42   2. 02   3. Application
   4. 5 = Implementation 5. Moderate

10. The nurse is instructing a client about a healthy diet. The nurse should instruct the client that the only essential fatty acid not synthesized by the body is linoleic acid and this can be obtained by eating foods such as

*A. sunflower oil.
B. margarine.
C. animal fat.
D. butter.

Reference: p. 1157

Descriptors: 1. 42   2. 02   3. Application
            4. 5 = Implementation 5. Moderate

11. An adult client tells the nurse that he needs to increase his intake of water-soluble vitamins. The nurse assesses the client to determine if he likes

A. fortified milk.
B. wheat germ.
C. sunflower oil.
*D. orange juice.

Reference: pp. 1158–1159

Descriptors: 1. 42   2. 03   3. Application
            4. 2 = Assessment   5. Moderate

12. The nurse is caring for a client who has been instructed about fat-soluble vitamins. The nurse determines that the client understands the instructions when she says she should eat foods such as

A. grapefruit juice.
B. seafood.
*C. fortified milk.
D. strawberries.

Reference: pp. 1158–1159

Descriptors: 1. 42   2. 03   3. Application
            4. 6 = Evaluation   5. Moderate

13. An adult client has been diagnosed with biliary disease. An important nutritional assessment for the nurse to make for this client is his intake of the vitamin

A. C.
B. B_{12}.
C. folate.
*D. A.

Reference: p. 1158

Descriptors: 1. 42   2. 04   3. Application
            4. 2 = Assessment   5. Moderate

14. A client with fatigue and pallor has been instructed by the nurse to consume foods that are high in folate. The nurse determines that the client understands the instructions when the nurse observes the client eating

A. scrambled eggs.
*B. spinach salad.
C. whole grapefruit.
D. broccoli.

Reference: p. 1159

Descriptors: 1. 42   2. 02   3. Application
            4. 6 = Evaluation   5. Moderate

15. The nurse is caring for a client who is on a fluid-restricted diet. The nurse should instruct the client that

A. large amounts of water are stored in the body.
B. most people have above-average fluid intake.
C. water intake averages about 1000 mL per day.
*D. solid foods may have a high water content.

Reference: p. 1158

Descriptors: 1. 42   2. 04   3. Application
            4. 5 = Implementation 5. Moderate

16. The nurse is caring for a client who complains of being thirsty and appears dehydrated. The nurse explains to the client that water loss can occur through urine, feces, perspiration, and

A. pancreatic secretions.
B. circulation.
*C. expired air.
D. metabolism.

Reference: p. 1158

Descriptors: 1. 42   2. 04   3. Application
            4. 5 = Implementation 5. Moderate

17. A client tells the nurse that she takes "lots of vitamins every day" but seems to be losing her hair. The nurse should assess the client's daily intake of

*A. vitamin A.
B. folate.
C. vitamin B_{12}.
D. biotin.

Reference: p. 1159

Descriptors: 1. 42   2. 02   3. Application
            4. 2 = Assessment   5. Moderate

18. A client visits the Urgent Care Center and tells the nurse he has had nausea and vomiting for 3 days and thinks he has the flu. The nurse should assess the client for symptoms of

A. adequate carbohydrate intake.
B. chronic fatigue.
C. vitamin C deficiency.
*D. dehydration.

Reference: p. 1158

Descriptors: 1. 42   2. 04   3. Application
            4. 2 = Assessment   5. Moderate

19. A client tells the nurse he needs to increase his intake of potassium. The nurse should instruct the client that a good source of potassium is

A. liver.
B. shellfish.
*C. bananas.
D. nuts.

Reference: p. 1160

Descriptors: 1. 42   2. 02   3. Application
        4. 5 = Implementation 5. Moderate

20. A client tells the nurse that he needs more copper in his diet. The nurse should assess whether the client likes

A. whole-grain bread.
*B. shellfish.
C. broccoli.
D. carrots.

Reference: p. 1160

Descriptors: 1. 42   2. 04   3. Application
        4. 2 = Assessment   5. Moderate

21. An adult client from Turkey is diagnosed with goiter. The nurse determines that the client's diet was most likely deficient in

A. potassium.
B. iron.
*C. iodine.
D. magnesium.

Reference: p. 1160

Descriptors: 1. 42   2. 04   3. Application
        4. 3 = Analysis/Diag.   5. Moderate

22. An adult female client tells the nurse that her fingernails are brittle and she is experiencing fatigue although she gets 10 hours of sleep per night. The nurse should assess the client's dietary intake of

*A. selenium.
B. chromium.
C. potassium.
D. sodium.

Reference: p. 1161

Descriptors: 1. 42   2. 04   3. Application
        4. 2 = Assessment   5. Moderate

23. The nurse has instructed a group of high school students about the Food Guide Pyramid. Following the instructions, the nurse determines that one of the students needs *further* instructions when she says,

A. "I should eat the minimum number of servings from the lower five groups."
B. "A serving size of meat equals 2 to 3 ounces of cooked meat."
*C. "Foods at the top of the pyramid should be eaten the most."
D. "One serving of bread is equal to one slice."

Reference: p. 1162

Descriptors: 1. 42   2. 03   3. Application
        4. 6 = Evaluation   5. Moderate

24. A 65-year-old male client who lives alone tells the nurse that he needs to decrease his sodium intake but doesn't know how to tell how much sodium is actually in the food he purchases. The nurse should instruct the client to

A. use a nutrition guide.
*B. read the product labels.
C. check the RDA chart.
D. follow the Food Guide Pyramid.

Reference: p. 1163

Descriptors: 1. 42   2. 02   3. Application
        4. 5 = Implementation 5. Moderate

25. The nurse plans to discuss nutritional needs with a group of adult clients. Which of the following would be important to include in the teaching plan?

A. Adult women should have an intake of 500 mg of calcium daily.
B. Adult men have higher iron requirements than women.
C. Adult women require a greater number of calories than men.
*D. Adult men require higher protein and vitamin B intake than women.

Reference: p. 1163

Descriptors: 1. 42   2. 05   3. Application
        4. 4 = Planning   5. Moderate

26. An adult client with moderate obesity is taking prescription medications for hypertension and he tells the nurse he suffers from constipation. The nurse should suggest to the client that he

A. chew his food thoroughly.
B. avoid cold liquids.
C. eat foods that are soft.
*D. increase his fluid intake.

Reference: p. 1165

Descriptors: 1. 42   2. 05   3. Application
        4. 5 = Implementation 5. Moderate

27. The nurse is caring for a client who has been diagnosed with hypoglycemia. The nurse should instruct the client to

   A. increase protein intake.
   B. eat 6 to 8 small meals daily.
  *C. avoid sugar-rich foods.
   D. take a multivitamin supplement.

Reference: p. 1165

Descriptors: 1. 42   2. 09   3. Application
          4. 5 = Implementation 5. Moderate

28. A new mother tells the nurse that the only way she can get her 4-week-old infant to sleep is to feed the infant oatmeal with his formula at night. The nurse should instruct the mother that

   A. a variety of cereals are necessary for good nutrition.
   B. strained vegetables would provide better nutrients than oatmeal.
   C. the oatmeal will provide the infant with necessary iron intake.
  *D. starch digestion does not develop until the age of 3 months.

Reference: p. 1166

Descriptors: 1. 42   2. 05   3. Application
          4. 5 = Implementation 5. Moderate

29. A client tells the nurse that her 15-month-old child has developed erratic eating patterns and frequently goes on a food jag requesting only peanut butter and jelly sandwiches. The nurse should instruct the client that the child

  *A. is exhibiting normal behavior for this age group.
   B. needs to have nutritional counseling.
   C. may not be receiving adequate protein.
   D. will develop poor nutritional habits later in life.

Reference: p. 1166

Descriptors: 1. 42   2. 05   3. Application
          4. 5 = Implementation 5. Moderate

30. The nurse is planning to conduct a nutrition class for a group of parents with school-age children. Which of the following would be important to include in the teaching plan?

   A. Children of this age group have a dramatic decrease in their appetites.
  *B. Fluoride, vitamins A and D, and calcium are important for dental health.
   C. Nutrient needs decrease towards the end of the school-age period.
   D. Food attitudes develop during this period of childhood.

Reference: p. 1166

Descriptors: 1. 42   2. 05   3. Application
          4. 4 = Planning   5. Moderate

31. The nurse is counseling a group of adolescents about nutritional needs during the adolescent period. The nurse should instruct the group that

   A. one in five teenage girls suffers from anorexia nervosa.
   B. iron needs increase, particularly for males, during adolescence.
  *C. physiologic age is a more valid indicator of need than chronological age.
   D. an estimated 1 in 100 girls experiences bulimia.

Reference: p. 1167

Descriptors: 1. 42   2. 05   3. Application
          4. 5 = Implementation 5. Moderate

32. The nurse is caring for a client who has just learned that she is approximately 8 weeks pregnant. Which of the following would be important for the nurse to include when counseling the client about nutritional needs during pregnancy? During pregnancy,

   A. a weight gain of 6 to 8 pounds during the first trimester is recommended.
  *B. iron and folic acid supplements are usually necessary.
   C. the amount of weight gained is more important than the pattern of weight gain.
   D. key nutrients include carbohydrates and vitamin D.

Reference: p. 1167

Descriptors: 1. 42   2. 05   3. Application
          4. 5 = Implementation 5. Moderate

33. The nurse is caring for an alert 79-year-old client who appears to have a decreased appetite and refuses to eat any meat. The nurse should assess the client for symptoms of

   A. gastrointestinal distress.
   B. constipation.
   C. metabolic disorders.
  *D. periodontal or jaw disease.

Reference: p. 1168

Descriptors: 1. 42   2. 05   3. Application
          4. 2 = Assessment   5. Moderate

34. The nurse makes a home visit to an 84-year-old client who is being cared for by her daughter. The daughter tells the nurse that she is concerned because her mother uses a large amount of salt on all of her food. The nurse should explain to the daughter that

  *A. as people age, the taste threshold for sugar and salt increases.
  B. the client may develop hypertension if salt intake is not decreased.
  C. salt should be removed from the client's dietary intake.
  D. excessive salt intake may lead to dehydration.

Reference: p. 1168

Descriptors: 1. 42   2. 05   3. Application
           4. 5 = Implementation 5. Moderate

35. The nurse is caring for an adult client who practices Orthodox Judaism and adheres to a kosher diet and needs additional protein. While assisting the client with her diet, the nurse recommends that the client consume more

  A. pork loin.
  B. crab meat.
  C. shrimp.
  *D. roast beef.

Reference: p. 1169

Descriptors: 1. 42   2. 08   3. Application
           4. 5 = Implementation 5. Moderate

36. A 16-year-old girl visits the clinic with her mother because the client has developed bizarre eating patterns and denies any appetite. The nurse determines that the client is most likely experiencing

  A. bulimia.
  B. yo-yo dieting.
  *C. anorexia nervosa.
  D. normal adolescent rebellion.

Reference: p. 1169

Descriptors: 1. 42   2. 05   3. Application
           4. 3 = Analysis/Diag. 5. Moderate

37. The nurse is caring for a client who has recently moved to the United States from Italy. The nurse should assess the client for a dietary deficiency of

  *A. calcium.
  B. protein.
  C. vitamin C.
  D. carbohydrates.

Reference: p. 1170

Descriptors: 1. 42   2. 07   3. Application
           4. 2 = Assessment 5. Moderate

38. The nurse is caring for a hospitalized postoperative client from Greece who has just been ordered a regular diet. While assisting the client to complete his diet menu, the nurse should suggest that the client choose

  A. a chocolate milk shake.
  *B. broiled lamb chops.
  C. spaghetti with meat sauce.
  D. stuffed grape leaves.

Reference: p. 1170

Descriptors: 1. 42   2. 08   3. Application
           4. 5 = Implementation 5. Moderate

39. An obese client visits the clinic and expresses a desire to be placed on a weight loss program. The best way for the nurse to collect dietary data on the client is to ask the client to

  A. provide a 24-hour recall of all food consumed.
  B. ask the client about food likes and dislikes.
  C. determine if the client takes vitamin and mineral supplements.
  *D. keep a food diary for 3 to 7 days.

Reference: p. 1172

Descriptors: 1. 42   2. 08   3. Application
           4. 5 = Implementation 5. Moderate

40. The nurse makes a home visit to a 76-year-old postoperative client who tells the nurse that she has "lost a lot of weight since the surgery." To obtain anthropometric data from the client, the nurse should

  *A. measure skin folds from several body sites.
  B. ask the client to recall foods consumed over the last 24 hours.
  C. determine if the client consumes adequate protein.
  D. gather information about medication usage.

Reference: pp. 1172, 1174

Descriptors: 1. 42   2. 06   3. Application
           4. 2 = Assessment 5. Moderate

41. An obese male client diagnosed with hypertension has been placed on a 1200 calorie low-fat diet. The client asks the nurse to tell him about what kinds of foods his wife should cook. A priority nursing diagnosis for this client is

  A. alteration in nutrition, more than body requirements related to poor metabolism.
  B. altered health maintenance related to change in normal dietary pattern.
  *C. knowledge deficit related to lack of information about low-fat foods.
  D. obesity related to inappropriate eating patterns and decreased activity.

Reference: p. 1176

Descriptors: 1. 42   2. 07   3. Application
           4. 3 = Analysis/Diag. 5. Moderate

42. A 38-year-old client visits the clinic 4 weeks after being placed on a weight reduction and exercise program. The client has gained 2 pounds since the last visit. She tells the nurse that she enjoys eating and frequently goes out with her friends for lunch. The client admits to exercising infrequently. A priority nursing diagnosis for this client is

   *A. noncompliance with low calorie diet and exercise program related to lack of motivation.
   B. knowledge deficit related to lack of interest in appropriate nutrition and need for exercise.
   C. altered nutrition, more than body requirements related to inability to maintain proper weight.
   D. altered nutrition related to overeating and lack of exercise in daily activities.

   Reference: p. 1176

   Descriptors: 1. 42   2. 07   3. Application
                4. 3 = Analysis/Diag.   5. Moderate

43. A 24-year-old client tells the nurse that she has been on a diet for the last 3 weeks and lately has become very fatigued when walking from the parking lot to her office. A laboratory value that the nurse should assess is the client's

   A. blood urea nitrogen.
   B. serum albumin.
   *C. hemoglobin.
   D. total lymphocyte count.

   Reference: p. 1178

   Descriptors: 1. 42   2. 09   3. Application
                4. 2 = Assessment   5. Moderate

44. A 32-year-old client visits the clinic and tells the nurse that although she has been on a 1200 calorie diet for the last month, she continues to gain weight. The client also complains of fatigue, dry skin, and amenorrhea. The nurse suspects the client may be experiencing a deficiency of

   A. serum albumin.
   *B. serum thyroxine.
   C. pancreatic enzyme.
   D. serum bilirubin.

   Reference: p. 1178

   Descriptors: 1. 42   2. 04   3. Interpretive
                4. 3 = Analysis/Diag.   5. Moderate

45. The nurse is caring for a postoperative client following bowel surgery when the client tells the nurse that she has had several frothy stools and has lost 10 pounds following the surgery. The client appears fatigued and malnourished. An important laboratory value for the nurse to assess is the client's

   A. basal metabolic rate.
   B. serum thyroxine.
   C. serum magnesium.
   *D. serum albumin.

   Reference: p. 1178

   Descriptors: 1. 42   2. 04   3. Application
                4. 3 = Analysis/Diag.   5. Moderate

46. After instructing a client and his wife about low-fat, low-calorie foods, the nurse determines that the client has understood the instructions when he says,

   A. "I should avoid drinking all beverages with caffeine."
   *B. "I shouldn't eat sandwiches made with processed meats."
   C. "A granola bar once a day is acceptable for a snack."
   D. "I should eat fruit at least once a day."

   Reference: pp. 1162, 1179

   Descriptors: 1. 42   2. 06   3. Application
                4. 6 = Evaluation   5. Moderate

47. The nurse visits a 78-year-old client whose husband is caring for the client following abdominal surgery. The husband tells the nurse that his wife has a poor appetite and seems to be losing weight. After giving suggestions for stimulating the client's appetite, the nurse determines that the husband needs *further* instructions when he says,

   *A. "It doesn't matter what the food looks like, as long as it tastes good."
   B. "It's important to offer alternatives if she doesn't like what I've served her."
   C. "I should avoid giving her medications just prior to a meal."
   D. "Small, frequent meals may be better than three large meals."

   Reference: p. 1179

   Descriptors: 1. 42   2. 09   3. Application
                4. 6 = Evaluation   5. Moderate

48. The nurse is caring for a 92-year-old client in a nursing home when the client appears to have a decreased appetite and a 5 pound weight loss. The client's serum albumin level is 33 g/L. The nurse should assess the client for

    A. anemia.
    B. jaundice.
    C. depression.
  *D. pressure ulcers.

Reference: p. 1180

Descriptors: 1. 42   2. 09   3. Application
            4. 2 = Assessment   5. Moderate

49. An adult client hospitalized following cardiac surgery has been instructed about a clear liquid diet. The nurse determines that the client understands the instructions when the client says he can have

    A. milk shakes.
    B. orange juice.
  *C. cherry Jello.
    D. creamed soups.

Reference: p. 1181

Descriptors: 1. 42   2. 09   3. Application
            4. 6 = Evaluation   5. Moderate

50. The nurse visits a client at home who will be on a full liquid diet for 7 days following abdominal surgery. The nurse should suggest to the client that he increase his intake of

    A. pureed vegetables.
    B. ground meats.
    C. sliced oranges.
  *D. protein supplements.

Reference: p. 1181

Descriptors: 1. 42   2. 07   3. Application
            4. 5 = Implementation 5. Moderate

51. A client tells the nurse that she is a vegetarian and asks whether additional vitamins are necessary. The nurse should instruct the client that she may need to supplement the vegetarian diet with

  *A. iron.
    B. zinc.
    C. calcium.
    D. vitamin C.

Reference: p. 1181

Descriptors: 1. 42   2. 08   3. Application
            4. 5 = Implementation 5. Moderate

52. The nurse has instructed a client about nasal intestinal tube feedings which the client will have following surgery. The nurse determines that the client understands the instructions when the client says,

    A. "This type of feeding is appropriate if I don't have any appetite."
    B. "Nasal intestinal tube feedings can result in aspiration."
  *C. "Dumping syndrome may occur with this type of feeding."
    D. "I may develop hyperglycemia with this type of feeding."

Reference: p. 1181

Descriptors: 1. 42   2. 09   3. Application
            4. 6 = Evaluation   5. Moderate

53. The nurse is caring for a client who has a nasogastric tube for intermittent feedings. Before beginning the next feeding the nurse plans to

    A. prepare the client for an x-ray examination.
  *B. measure the pH of the stomach aspirate.
    C. remove air from the tube.
    D. flush the tube with water.

Reference: pp. 1182, 1186

Descriptors: 1. 42   2. 08   3. Application
            4. 4 = Planning   5. Moderate

54. The nurse is preparing to insert a rubber nasogastric tube into an adult client. Before beginning the insertion the nurse should

    A. position the client in a semi-Fowler's position.
    B. measure the distance from the client's nostril to the xyphoid process.
    C. don sterile gloves after opening the tube package.
  *D. place the tube in a basin with ice for 5 to 10 minutes.

Reference: p. 1183

Descriptors: 1. 42   2. 08   3. Application
            4. 5 = Implementation 5. Moderate

55. While inserting a nasogastric tube into an adult client, the client begins to gag. The nurse should

    A. instruct the client to take deep breaths for several minutes.
  *B. check the tube position with a tongue blade and flashlight.
    C. discontinue the procedure and remove the tube.
    D. ask the client to hold his head and neck in a hyperextended position.

Reference: p. 1184

Descriptors: 1. 42   2. 08   3. Application
            4. 5 = Implementation 5. Moderate

56. The nurse is caring for a client with nasogastric tube feedings. After several attempts to aspirate GI fluid from the tube with a syringe, the nurse has been unsuccessful in obtaining fluid. The nurse should

  A. remove the tube and reinsert a new nasogastric tube.
  B. flush the tube with 50 mL of water
  *C. change the client's position and raise the head of the bed.
  D. instill air and leave the large syringe in place for 1 hour.

Reference: p. 1186

Descriptors: 1. 42   2. 08   3. Application
            4. 5 = Implementation 5. Moderate

57. The nurse is caring for a client who is receiving intermittent feedings through a nasogastric tube. The nurse has aspirated the gastric contents and measured 110 mL of residual fluid. The nurse should

  *A. report these findings to the client's physician.
  B. inform the oncoming nurse during the shift report.
  C. dispose of the gastric contents in the client's commode.
  D. flush the tube with 110 mL of sterile water.

Reference: p. 1188

Descriptors: 1. 42   2. 08   3. Application
            4. 5 = Implementation 5. Moderate

58. The nurse is caring for a client who is receiving continuous feedings through a nasogastric tube. While caring for this client the nurse plans to

  A. hang the feeding solution 16 inches above the client's stomach.
  *B. check the residual every 4 to 8 hours.
  C. ask the client to remain in a supine position for 1 hour after the feeding.
  D. assess for bowel sounds every 2 hours.

Reference: pp. 1188, 1189–1191

Descriptors: 1. 42   2. 09   3. Application
            4. 4 = Planning   5. Moderate

59. The nurse has instructed a caregiver of a client how to administer tube feedings through a jejunostomy tube. The nurse determines that the caregiver needs *further* instructions when the caregiver says,

  A. "I should refrigerate the formula and discard it after 24 hours."
  *B. "If the skin around the area becomes reddened, I should cleanse the area."
  C. "I should change the delivery set every 24 hours using aseptic technique."
  D. "I should flush the tube with water before and after feeding."

Reference: p. 1191

Descriptors: 1. 42   2. 09   3. Application
            4. 6 = Evaluation   5. Moderate

60. When the nurse prepares to remove a nasogastric feeding tube from an adult client, the nurse should

  *A. instruct the client to take a deep breath and hold it.
  B. don sterile gloves before beginning the procedure.
  C. inject 50 mL of normal saline to clear the tube.
  D. remove the tube slowly while the client exhales deeply.

Reference: p. 1194

Descriptors: 1. 42   2. 09   3. Application
            4. 5 = Implementation 5. Moderate

61. The nurse is caring for a hospitalized client who has a Salem sump tube in place for decompression following surgery. The nurse plans to

  A. irrigate the tube with 30 mL of sterile water every 4 hours.
  B. remove 30 mL of air from the air vent on the tube.
  *C. irrigate the tube with 30 mL of normal saline every 4 hours.
  D. position the client in a side-lying position.

Reference: pp. 1193, 1195

Descriptors: 1. 42   2. 08   3. Application
            4. 4 = Planning   5. Moderate

62. The nurse is caring for a client who will be receiving parenteral nutrition through a central vein for several weeks. The nurse plans to

  A. weigh the client once a week.
  *B. monitor serum protein levels daily.
  C. assess blood glucose levels every 24 hours.
  D. assess the client for symptoms of hypercalcemia.

Reference: pp. 1193, 1196

Descriptors: 1. 42   2. 10   3. Application
            4. 4 = Planning   5. Moderate

63. The nurse has instructed a moderately obese client about a weight loss program. The client will be receiving a 1200 calorie daily diet. The nurse determines that the client needs *further* instructions when he says,

  A. "I should keep low-calorie foods towards the front of the refrigerator."
  *B. "It's important to try to lose at least 4 to 5 pounds per week."
  C. "I shouldn't weigh myself too often."
  D. "I should wait 10 minutes after feeling the urge to eat."

Reference: p. 1202

Descriptors: 1. 42   2. 09   3. Application
            4. 6 = Evaluation   5. Moderate

64. A client who has been diagnosed with iron-deficiency anemia asks the nurse how to improve her hemoglobin levels. The nurse should instruct the client to

A. eat a source of heme iron at least once per day.
B. include a rich source of calcium with every meal.
C. drink a cup of hot tea with every meal.
*D. eat citrus fruits or cantaloupe with every meal.

Reference: p. 1201

Descriptors: 1. 42   2. 08   3. Application
              4. 5 = Implementation 5. Moderate

65. A young mother tells the nurse that her 3-year-old son consumes 1 to 2 quarts of milk daily and is a "finicky eater." The nurse should assess the toddler for

A. malabsorption syndrome.
B. chronic diarrhea.
C. malnutrition.
*D. iron-deficiency anemia.

Reference: p. 1201

Descriptors: 1. 42   2. 04   3. Application
              4. 2 = Assessment   5. Moderate

CHAPTER 43
Urinary Elimination

1. As urine collects in the bladder, the desire to void is experienced due to stimulation of the

A. sympathetic nervous system.
B. nephrons in the kidney.
*C. stretch receptors.
D. external sphincter.

Reference: p. 1213

Descriptors: 1. 43   2. 02   3. Factual
              4. 1 = No Process   5. Moderate

2. An adult client tells the nurse that she is "very embarrassed and just not able" to obtain a requested urine sample. The nurse determines that the client's inability to obtain the sample is due to

A. urinary retention related to the aging process.
B. decreased amount of abdominal pressure.
*C. inability to relax the restraining muscles of the bladder.
D. loss of muscle tone in the bladder.

Reference: p. 1213

Descriptors: 1. 43   2. 02   3. Application
              4. 3 = Analysis/Diag. 5. Moderate

3. An adult client tells the nurse that she voids frequently in small amounts and has done this most of her life. The nurse determines that the client is most likely experiencing

A. urinary incontinence.
*B. a normal pattern of voiding.
C. decreased bladder control.
D. urinary retention.

Reference: p. 1214

Descriptors: 1. 43   2. 02   3. Application
              4. 3 = Analysis/Diag. 5. Moderate

4. A new mother tells the nurse that she is concerned because her 13-month-old infant still uses diapers and will not use the potty chair to void. The nurse should instruct the mother that

*A. most children begin to control urination voluntarily at 18 to 24 months.
B. the mother should keep trying by placing the child on the potty chair at frequent intervals.
C. the child may need further evaluation by a medical specialist.
D. lifelong attitudes about voiding begin at 12 months of age.

Reference: p. 1214

Descriptors: 1. 43   2. 02   3. Application
              4. 5 = Implementation 5. Moderate

5. The nurse has instructed a caregiver of a 79-year-old client with occasional urinary incontinence about the effects of aging on urination patterns. The nurse determines that the caregiver needs *further* instructions when the caregiver says,

A. "Decreased bladder muscle tone may result in increased frequency."
B. "Neuromuscular problems and weakness may interfere with voluntary control."
C. "Decreased ability of the kidneys to concentrate urine may result in nocturia."
*D. Increased bladder contractility may lead to urinary incontinence."

Reference: p. 1214

Descriptors: 1. 43   2. 03   3. Application
              4. 6 = Evaluation   5. Moderate

6. The nurse is planning to obtain a urine specimen from a dehydrated client with a fever of 100.4°F. The nurse anticipates that the urine will be

A. discolored.
B. diluted.
C. frothy.
*D. concentrated.

Reference: pp. 1214, 1216

Descriptors: 1. 43   2. 03   3. Application
              4. 2 = Assessment   5. Moderate

7. A client tells the nurse that he voids frequently throughout the day and must get out of bed at night to void. The nurse should assess the client's dietary consumption of

A. potato chips.
B. lemonade.
*C. coffee.
D. milk.

Reference: p. 1214

Descriptors: 1. 43   2. 03   3. Application
        4. 2 = Assessment   5. Moderate

8. The nurse makes a home visit to a 75-year-old client who is moderately immobile due to arthritis. While assessing the client's urinary elimination patterns the nurse should pay particular attention to symptoms of

A. urinary frequency.
*B. urinary stasis.
C. bladder spasms.
D. kidney disorders.

Reference: p. 1215

Descriptors: 1. 43   2. 03   3. Application
        4. 2 = Assessment   5. Moderate

9. An adult client has been given a prescription for oral Pyridium as a urinary tract analgesic. The nurse should instruct the client that the medication may cause

A. hematuria.
B. greenish-colored urine.
C. urinary retention.
*D. orange-colored urine.

Reference: p. 1216

Descriptors: 1. 43   2. 03   3. Application
        4. 5 = Implementation   5. Moderate

10. An adult female client visits the clinic and tells the nurse that the color of her urine is blue. The nurse should assess the client for

*A. intake of B-complex vitamins.
B. use of analgesic medications.
C. consumption of iron compounds.
D. frequency of douching.

Reference: p. 1216

Descriptors: 1. 43   2. 03   3. Application
        4. 2 = Assessment   5. Moderate

11. A group of adults is planning a 6-hour bus trip throughout the state. The nurse should suggest that the best fluid they could take on the trip is

*A. water.
B. colas.
C. fruit punch.
D. iced tea.

Reference: p. 1216

Descriptors: 1. 43   2. 03   3. Application
        4. 5 = Implementation   5. Moderate

12. While performing a physical examination of an adult client, the nurse should assess the client's kidneys by

A. gently tapping the flank area with two fingers.
*B. deeply palpating while under supervision.
C. moderately palpating the costovertebral angle.
D. using the dominant hand to palpate the abdominal wall.

Reference: p. 1217

Descriptors: 1. 43   2. 04   3. Application
        4. 5 = Implementation   5. Moderate

13. While percussing an adult client's bladder above the symphysis pubis, the nurse notes a dull sound. The nurse determines that the client is most likely experiencing a/an

*A. full bladder.
B. empty bladder.
C. urinary retention.
D. urinary infection.

Reference: p. 1217

Descriptors: 1. 43   2. 04   3. Application
        4. 3 = Analysis/Diag.   5. Moderate

14. After an adult client has voided, the nurse assesses the client's bladder and would normally find that the bladder is

A. above the symphysis pubis.
B. smooth to the touch.
*C. unable to be palpated.
D. tender to touch.

Reference: p. 1217

Descriptors: 1. 43   2. 04   3. Application
        4. 2 = Assessment   5. Moderate

15. To obtain a urine sample for a routine urinalysis from an adult client who has voided into a bedpan, the nurse should

*A. wear clean gloves.
B. place the specimen on ice.
C. measure the amount in the specimen container.
D. wear sterile gloves.

Reference: p. 1218

Descriptors: 1. 43   2. 04   3. Application
        4. 5 = Implementation   5. Easy

16. A postoperative adult client with an indwelling catheter needs to have his urine output measured hourly. After measuring the amount of urine produced during the last hour, the nurse should

    A. empty the urine into the client's toilet while wearing gloves.
    B. notify the physician if the amount of urine is less than 100 mL.
    C. leave the urine in the calibrated measuring chamber until it is full.
  *D. tilt the measuring chamber and allow the urine to enter the collection bag.

Reference: p. 1219

Descriptors: 1. 43   2. 05   3. Application
            4. 5 = Implementation 5. Moderate

17. An adult hospitalized client tells the nurse that during the last two voidings he has experienced pain and burning. The nurse should notify the physician of the client's

  *A. dysuria.
    B. polyuria.
    C. pyuria.
    D. nocturia

Reference: p. 1219

Descriptors: 1. 43   2. 01   3. Application
            4. 3 = Analysis/Diag. 5. Moderate

18. The nurse is caring for an adult client whose urine output was 400 mL during the last 24 hours. The nurse documents the client's

    A. urinary retention.
    B. pneumaturia.
    C. pyuria.
  *D. oliguria.

Reference: p. 1219

Descriptors: 1. 43   2. 01   3. Application
            4. 2 = Assessment 5. Moderate

19. The nurse plans to collect a urine specimen for a routine urinalysis from an alert adult client. The nurse plans to obtain a

  *A. clean container.
    B. sterile container.
    C. sterile bedpan.
    D. clean catheter.

Reference: p. 1220

Descriptors: 1. 43   2. 05   3. Application
            4. 4 = Planning   5. Moderate

20. The nurse obtains a straw-colored, clear urine sample from an adult client and determines that the urine pH is 6.0 with a specific gravity of 1.020. The nurse determines that the client's urine most likely indicates

    A. overhydration.
    B. underhydration.
    C. infection.
  *D. normal findings.

Reference: p. 1220

Descriptors: 1. 43   2. 05   3. Application
            4. 3 = Analysis/Diag. 5. Moderate

21. An adult client who is very athletic and eats a high-protein diet daily obtains a urine sample for the nurse. The nurse anticipates that because of the high protein intake, the client's urine will likely be

    A. cloudy.
  *B. acidic.
    C. alkaline.
    D. sulfuric.

Reference: p. 1220

Descriptors: 1. 43   2. 05   3. Application
            4. 3 = Analysis/Diag. 5. Moderate

22. The nurse requests an adult male client to obtain an ordered clean-catch urine specimen. The nurse should instruct the client to

  *A. collect the urine in a sterile container.
    B. void first, then collect the specimen 30 minutes later.
    C. use a clean container to collect 100 mL of urine.
    D. cleanse the meatus with alcohol before voiding.

Reference: pp. 1220–1221

Descriptors: 1. 43   2. 05   3. Application
            4. 5 = Implementation 5. Moderate

23. The nurse is planning to collect a clean-catch specimen from a female client on bedrest when the client says "I don't think I can void into the container." The nurse plans to ask the client to

    A. void into a bedside commode and then pour 30 mL into the container.
  *B. use a sterile bedpan to collect the specimen and transfer it to a container.
    C. discard the first 100 mL of urine and collect the remainder.
    D. collect all urine into a clean bedpan, then measure 30 m. for a specimen.

Reference: p. 1222

Descriptors: 1. 43   2. 05   3. Application
            4. 4 = Planning   5. Moderate

24. The nurse is preparing to collect a urine specimen for routine urinalysis from an adult client with an indwelling catheter. The nurse should

  A. clamp the tube below the collection port for 60 minutes.
  B. collect at least 10 mL of urine from the collection bag.
  C. use sterile gloves to obtain the urine.
  *D. withdraw the urine with a syringe from the port in the catheter.

  Reference: p. 1223

  Descriptors: 1. 43   2. 05   3. Application
              4. 5 = Implementation 5. Moderate

25. The physician has ordered a 24-hour urine collection for an adult client. The nurse begins the collection procedure at 6 AM by

  A. starting a new intake and output flowsheet.
  *B. asking the client to void and discard the specimen.
  C. putting a sign on the client's bed.
  D. placing the collection container in a pan of ice.

  Reference: p. 1223

  Descriptors: 1. 43   2. 05   3. Application
              4. 5 = Implementation 5. Moderate

26. A home care client is to have his urine tested for protein using plastic strips with a special coating. The nurse should instruct the client that when the color of the strip changes after contact with the urine, this is due to the strip's

  A. preservative.
  B. alkalinity.
  *C. reagent.
  D. acidity.

  Reference: p. 1224

  Descriptors: 1. 43   2. 05   3. Application
              4. 5 = Implementation 5. Moderate

27. When using a hydrometer to assess the specific gravity of a client's urine, the nurse should

  *A. read the measurement at eye level at the bottom of the meniscus.
  B. shake the hydrometer briefly before taking the measurement.
  C. hold the hydrometer above eye level and read above the meniscus.
  D. allow 15 minutes before taking the measurement to allow time for the reagent.

  Reference: p. 1224

  Descriptors: 1. 43   2. 05   3. Application
              4. 5 = Implementation 5. Moderate

28. The nurse is caring for a 66-year-old client at home when the client tells the nurse that she is "afraid to go anywhere because I often lose my urine." A priority nursing diagnosis for this client is

  A. risk for skin breakdown related to urinary incontinence.
  B. potential for sleep pattern disturbance related to nocturia.
  C. toileting self-care deficit related to urinary frequency.
  *D. self-esteem disturbance related to urinary incontinence.

  Reference: p. 1225

  Descriptors: 1. 43   2. 06   3. Application
              4. 3 = Analysis/Diag. 5. Moderate

29. The nurse is caring for a postoperative client with an indwelling catheter who is on a clear liquid diet. An appropriate goal for the client's urinary elimination pattern is that the client will

  *A. produce urine output about equal to fluid intake.
  B. void within 2 hours after removal of the indwelling catheter.
  C. maintain an alkaline pH of the urine.
  D. report any incontinence of urine to the nursing staff.

  Reference: p. 1225

  Descriptors: 1. 43   2. 05   3. Application
              4. 4 = Planning   5. Moderate

30. An adult client is scheduled for a cystoscopy in the morning. The nurse should instruct the client that she will

  A. remain NPO after midnight.
  B. be monitored for urinary frequency after the procedure.
  *C. need to sign an informed consent statement before the procedure.
  D. be given pain medication after the procedure is completed.

  Reference: p. 1226

  Descriptors: 1. 43   2. 05   3. Application
              4. 5 = Implementation 5. Moderate

31. The nurse has instructed an alert adult client about intravenous pyelography which is scheduled the next day. The nurse determines that the client understands the instructions when the client says,

  *A. "I will need to void before the examination."
  B. "No preparation is needed for this procedure."
  C. "I can maintain my normal eating patterns before the procedure."
  D. "There are no side effects from this procedure."

  Reference: p. 1226

  Descriptors: 1. 43   2. 05   3. Application
              4. 6 = Evaluation   5. Moderate

32. An adult client hospitalized following an automobile accident is scheduled for a retrograde pyelography examination in the morning. The nurse should plan to

   A. provide the client with a clear liquid breakfast in the morning.
   B. ask the client not to void the morning of the examination.
   *C. give the client an ordered laxative the evening before the examination.
   D. administer an ordered analgesic the evening before the examination.

   Reference: p. 1226

   Descriptors: 1. 43   2. 05   3. Application
                4. 4 = Planning   5. Moderate

33. An adult client is scheduled for an ultrasound of her kidneys on the following day. Following instructions about the procedure, the nurse determines that the client needs *further* instructions when the client says,

   *A. "It is alright for me to chew gum before the procedure."
   B. "This procedure is painless."
   C. "I will need to sign a consent form before the procedure."
   D. "The results of the test are usually ready 1 to 2 days after the procedure."

   Reference: p. 1226

   Descriptors: 1. 43   2. 05   3. Application
                4. 6 = Evaluation   5. Moderate

34. An adult client is scheduled for a computerized tomography of his bladder and a contrast dye is to be used. The nurse should

   A. keep the client NPO for 12 hours before the test.
   B. withhold any prescribed medications usually taken.
   C. tape the client's wedding rings in place.
   *D. assess the client for history of an allergic reaction to shellfish.

   Reference: p. 1226

   Descriptors: 1. 43   2. 05   3. Application
                4. 2 = Assessment   5. Moderate

35. The nurse is caring for a hospitalized 4-year-old who has been wetting his bed since his admission. The mother tells the nurse that the child has been toilet-trained for over a year. The nurse determines that the client is most likely experiencing

   A. stress incontinence.
   *B. functional incontinence.
   C. urinary tract infection.
   D. urinary retention with overflow.

   Reference: p. 1227

   Descriptors: 1. 43   2. 06   3. Interpretive
                4. 3 = Analysis/Diag.   5. Moderate

36. An obese client with three children tells the nurse that when she laughs suddenly, she dribbles urine down the side of her leg. The nurse suspects that the client is experiencing

   A. urge incontinence.
   B. urinary retention.
   *C. stress incontinence.
   D. reflex relaxation.

   Reference: p. 1227

   Descriptors: 1. 43   2. 06   3. Interpretive
                4. 3 = Analysis/Diag.   5. Moderate

37. The nurse makes a home visit to an 80-year-old client who tells the nurse that she has trouble making it to the bathroom in time and urinates before she gets there. The nurse determines that the client is experiencing

   A. nocturnal frequency.
   B. urinary retention.
   *C. urge incontinence.
   D. reflex incontinence.

   Reference: p. 1227

   Descriptors: 1. 43   2. 06   3. Interpretive
                4. 3 = Analysis/Diag.   5. Moderate

38. The nurse is assisting a postoperative male client to void. Besides providing the client with privacy, the nurse should

   *A. help the client assume a normal voiding position.
   B. turn the client to his dominant side before voiding.
   C. offer the client a bedside commode for voiding.
   D. stay near the client while he voids in the urinal.

   Reference: p. 1228

   Descriptors: 1. 43   2. 07   3. Application
                4. 5 = Implementation 5. Moderate

39. An adult client who is active in sports activities tells the nurse that she often dribbles her urine when she least expects it. The nurse should instruct the client to

   A. wear protective underwear.
   B. limit fluid intake while active.
   *C. practice Kegel exercises at least 30 times per day.
   D. decrease the number of sports activities.

   Reference: p. 1228

   Descriptors: 1. 43   2. 07   3. Application
                4. 5 = Implementation 5. Moderate

40. An adult client has been instructed about how to perform Kegel's exercises. The nurse determines that the client understands the instructions when she says,

   *A. "I should contract the pelvic floor muscles for 10 seconds."
   B. "It's important that I do the exercises at least once per week."
   C. "I need to do these exercises for the rest of my life."
   D. "I should contract and then relax the muscles for at least 20 to 30 seconds."

   Reference: p. 1228

   Descriptors: 1. 43   2. 05   3. Application
               4. 6 = Evaluation   5. Moderate

41. A female client tells the nurse that she sometimes experiences hesitancy when trying to void. After instructing the client about various methods to resolve this problem, the nurse determines that the client needs *further* instructions when the client says she should

   *A. use Crede's manuevers to stimulate a urine stream.
   B. pour warm water over her fingers while trying to void.
   C. void when the urge to void is first experienced.
   D. use warm water over the perineal area to stimulate voiding.

   Reference: p. 1228

   Descriptors: 1. 43   2. 07   3. Application
               4. 6 = Evaluation   5. Moderate

42. A caregiver of an 80-year-old client tells the nurse that her mother frequently experiences nocturia and is sometimes incontinent. Following instructions about strategies to resolve the elimination problems, the nurse determines that the caregiver understands the instructions when she says,

   A. "Soft slippers can prevent my mother from falling during the night."
   B. "I should be sure that my mother drinks at least 2500 mL of fluid before 5 PM."
   *C. "Beverages with caffeine and Nutrasweet should be avoided before bedtime."
   D. "My mother may need to have an indwelling catheter in place."

   Reference: p. 1229

   Descriptors: 1. 43   2. 07   3. Application
               4. 6 = Evaluation   5. Moderate

43. The nurse is assisting a female client on bedrest with perineal care following urination on a bedpan. Following instructions about the proper technique, the nurse determines that the client understands the instructions when the nurse observes the client clean the perineal area

   A. in a circular motion around the meatus.
   B. once a day with mild soap and water.
   *C. from front to back.
   D. from the back towards the front.

   Reference: p. 1230

   Descriptors: 1. 43   2. 07   3. Application
               4. 6 = Evaluation   5. Moderate

44. The nurse is preparing to assist a client on complete bedrest to use the bedpan for voiding. The nurse should *first*

   A. don sterile gloves.
   B. place the bed in the lowest position.
   *C. warm the bedpan if it is made of metal.
   D. be certain toilet tissue is available.

   Reference: p. 1232

   Descriptors: 1. 43   2. 05   3. Application
               4. 5 = Implementation 5. Moderate

45. After a client has voided, the nurse measures the client's post-void residual as 45 mL. The nurse determines that that the client is most likely experiencing

   *A. normal bladder function.
   B. stress incontinence.
   C. urinary retention.
   D. functional incontinence.

   Reference: p. 1234

   Descriptors: 1. 43   2. 08   3. Application
               4. 3 = Analysis/Diag.   5. Moderate

46. The nurse is caring for a postoperative client who has had frequent urinary incontinence since the client had surgery. The client's husband says, "Why don't the doctors just order a catheter for her?" The best response by the nurse is to instruct the client's husband that urinary catheters

   A. can affect the client's future voiding patterns.
   B. require an incision above the pubic area.
   C. affect the client's mobility patterns.
   *D. are the most prominent cause of nosocomial infections.

   Reference: p. 1235

   Descriptors: 1. 43   2. 07   3. Application
               4. 5 = Implementation 5. Moderate

47. The nurse makes a home visit to an adult client who has had a urologic stent inserted two days ago. While assessing the stent, the nurse observes that the urine from the stent is bright red in color. The nurse should

A. continue to monitor the output daily.
*B. notify the client's physician immediately.
C. irrigate the stent with sterile water.
D. measure the amount of urine output.

Reference: p. 1236

Descriptors: 1. 43   2. 07   3. Application
            4. 5 = Implementation 5. Moderate

48. The nurse is preparing to catheterize an 80-year-old client with arthritis and a left hip joint replacement. The nurse plans to position the client in which of the following positions?

*A. Sims
B. Dorsal recumbent
C. Lithotomy
D. Supine

Reference: p. 1237

Descriptors: 1. 43   2. 07   3. Application
            4. 4 = Planning   5. Moderate

49. The nurse is planning to insert an indwelling catheter in an adult male client. The nurse plans to

A. remove the catheter if pressure is felt by the client.
B. use an 8-French size catheter.
C. insert the catheter to 1 inch beyond the point where urine flows.
*D. insert the catheter to the bifurcation of the catheter tubing

Reference: p. 1237

Descriptors: 1. 43   2. 07   3. Application
            4. 4 = Planning   5. Moderate

50. The nurse is preparing to insert an indwelling catheter into an adult female client. Before inserting the catheter, the nurse should *first*

A. spread the labia with the dominant hand.
*B. test the catheter balloon for patency.
C. wear clean gloves to pour the antiseptic solution.
D. clean the meatus by moving the moistened cotton ball up from the rectum.

Reference: p. 1240

Descriptors: 1. 43   2. 07   3. Application
            4. 5 = Implementation 5. Moderate

51. A client has not voided for 8 hours and a straight catheterization is ordered. After removing 750 mL of urine through the catheter, the nurse stops the procedure in order to prevent the client from experiencing

A. a need for additional catheterizations at a later time.
*B. engorgement of pelvic floor muscles and hypotension.
C. further relaxation of the urethral sphincter.
D. irritability of the bladder muscle which may cause discomfort.

Reference: p. 1241

Descriptors: 1. 43   2. 07   3. Application
            4. 3 = Analysis/Diag.   5. Moderate

52. While performing a catheterization on an adult female client, there is not an immediate flow of urine from the catheter. The nurse should

A. obtain a larger-sized catheter for another catheterization.
B. remove the catheter and reinsert another catheter.
*C. rotate the catheter slightly while leaving it in place.
D. raise the foot of the client's bed.

Reference: p. 1243

Descriptors: 1. 43   2. 07   3. Application
            4. 5 = Implementation 5. Moderate

53. The nurse is preparing to give a continuous bladder irrigation to an adult male client. The nurse plans to

*A. hang the solution bag on a pole 2 to 3 feet above the client's bladder.
B. allow air from the solution bag tubing to flow into the catheter.
C. use aseptic technique to attach the solution bag tubing to the catheter.
D. clamp the tubing of the solution bag periodically to prevent bladder distention.

Reference: p. 1248

Descriptors: 1. 43   2. 07   3. Application
            4. 4 = Planning   5. Moderate

54. The nurse has instructed a caregiver of an adult client about care of the client with an indwelling catheter. The nurse determines that the caregiver understands the instructions when the nurse observes the caregiver

   A. use mild hand lotion around the labia to moisten the tissue.
   *B. wash the perineal area with soap and water at least twice daily.
   C. apply baby powder to the perineal area and thighs after cleansing.
   D. open the closed drainage system to measure the amount of urine.

   Reference: p. 1249

   Descriptors: 1. 43   2. 07   3. Application
               4. 6 = Evaluation   5. Moderate

55. The nurse is caring for an adult female client with an indwelling catheter. To help keep the urine acidic, the nurse suggests to the client that she drink

   A. iced tea.
   B. fruit punch.
   C. grape juice.
   *D. cranberry juice.

   Reference: p. 1249

   Descriptors: 1. 43   2. 07   3. Application
               4. 5 = Implementation 5. Moderate

56. The nurse is planning to remove an indwelling catheter from an adult male client. During the procedure, the nurse plans to

   A. cleanse the perineal area before removal of the catheter.
   B. measure the amount of urine in the catheter tubing.
   *C. aspirate the fluid in the inflated balloon.
   D. use sterile scissors to cut the tubing and deflate the balloon.

   Reference: p. 1250

   Descriptors: 1. 43   2. 07   3. Application
               4. 4 = Planning   5. Moderate

57. The nurse has instructed the client about care following the removal of an indwelling catheter. The nurse determines that the client needs *further* instructions when the client says,

   *A. "I need to keep track of my intake for the next 48 hours."
   B. "I should continue to drink plenty of fluids."
   C. "The first time or two that I void I might have a slight burning sensation."
   D. "I should tell the nurse if I see any blood in my urine when I void."

   Reference: p. 1250

   Descriptors: 1. 43   2. 07   3. Application
               4. 6 = Evaluation   5. Moderate

58. The nurse has instructed a home care client about self-catheterizations. The nurse determines that the client understands the instructions when she says,

   A. "I should plan to catheterize myself at least every 2 hours."
   *B. "I should drink at least 1 to 2 quarts of fluid daily."
   C. "The catheter should be washed with a bleach solution after use."
   D. "When the catheter is in place, I should press down on the meatus to fully empty the bladder."

   Reference: pp. 1250–1251

   Descriptors: 1. 43   2. 09   3. Application
               4. 6 = Evaluation   5. Moderate

59. The nurse is preparing to change a male client's condom catheter. The nurse plans to

   A. don sterile gloves before removing the previous condom catheter.
   B. keep the tip of the tubing 2 to 5 inches beyond the tip of the penis.
   *C. wash the penis after removal of the condom catheter and dry thoroughly.
   D. position the tubing of the new condom catheter close to the penis.

   Reference: p. 1251

   Descriptors: 1. 43   2. 07   3. Application
               4. 4 = Planning   5. Moderate

60. The nurse is caring for a client who has an ileal conduit following surgery. The nurse should instruct the client that

   A. fluid restriction is necessary since a limited amount of urine will be produced.
   *B. the appliance to collect urine should be emptied frequently throughout the day.
   C. the client will need assistance in voiding at least every 8 hours.
   D. no tub baths will be allowed, but the client can shower.

   Reference: p. 1251

   Descriptors: 1. 43   2. 07   3. Application
               4. 5 = Implementation 5. Moderate

61. A 25-year-old mother visits the clinic with her 5-year-old son and tells the nurse that her son has been wetting the bed for the past two weeks. Following instructions, about strategies to cope with the problem, the nurse determines that the mother needs *further* instructions when she says,

*A. "It's acceptable to punish him by limiting television after he wets the bed."
B. "He can keep a calendar with dry days and nights circled."
C. "He should outgrow the bed-wetting between the ages of 6 and 8 years."
D. "I should limit the fluid intake at night and have him void before bedtime."

Reference: p. 1256

Descriptors: 1. 43　　2. 09　　3. Application
　　　　　　4. 6 = Evaluation　5. Moderate

62. A 75-year-old male client tells the nurse that he has had a great deal of difficulty voiding during the past week. The nurse determines that the most likely reason for the client's urinary retention is a/an

*A. enlarged prostate gland.
B. urinary tract infection.
C. enlarged bladder capacity.
D. injury to the spinal cord.

Reference: p. 1256

Descriptors: 1. 43　　2. 09　　3. Application
　　　　　　4. 3 = Analysis/Diag.　5. Moderate

63. An adult client who has had urinary retention is given a prescription for bethanechol chloride (Urecholine). The nurse explains to the client that the drug

A. reduces swelling.
B. provides pain relief.
*C. stimulates micturation.
D. acidifies urine in the bladder.

Reference: p. 1257

Descriptors: 1. 43　　2. 09　　3. Application
　　　　　　4. 5 = Implementation 5. Moderate

64. The nurse is caring for a client with an indwelling catheter when the nurse observes that the client's urine culture shows 100,000/mL bacterial colonies. The nurse should

*A. notify the client's physician.
B. force fluids often to the client.
C. continue to monitor the client's output.
D. flush the catheter with normal saline.

Reference: p. 1257

Descriptors: 1. 43　　2. 09　　3. Application
　　　　　　4. 5 = Implementation 5. Moderate

CHAPTER 44
Bowel Elimination

1. The amount of chyme processed daily by the large intestine is about

A. 500 mL.
B. 1000 mL.
*C. 1500 mL.
D. 2000 mL.

Reference: p. 1266

Descriptors: 1. 44　　2. 02　　3. Factual
　　　　　　4. 1 = No Process　5. Easy

2. Functions of the human body's large intestine include finishing absorption, manufacturing of vitamins, formation of feces, and

A. fat storage.
*B. expulsion of feces.
C. digestion of lactose.
D. initiation of peristalsis.

Reference: p. 1266

Descriptors: 1. 44　　2. 02　　3. Factual
　　　　　　4. 1 = No Process　5. Easy

3. Vertical folds in the rectum each contain an artery and a vein. When the vein is abnormally distended, this results in

A. stricture.
B. diverticulis.
*C. hemorrhoids.
D. diarrhea.

Reference: p. 1267

Descriptors: 1. 44　　2. 01　　3. Factual
　　　　　　4. 1 = No Process　5. Easy

4. The nurse is caring for a first time mother who is breastfeeding her neonate. The nurse plans to instruct the client that stools of breastfed infants

A. are firm and yellow to brown in color.
B. are soft and dark brown in color.
C. usually average from 1 to 2 per day.
*D. usually average from 2 to 4 per day.

Reference: p. 1269

Descriptors: 1. 44　　2. 03　　3. Application
　　　　　　4. 4 = Planning　5. Moderate

5. A young mother visits the clinic with her 18-month-old son. The mother tells the nurse that no matter what she does, the child just isn't interested in using the potty chair for a bowel movement. The nurse should instruct the mother that

   A. she should continue working with the child on potty training.
   B. she should schedule an appointment for a comprehensive evaluation.
   C. it is possible that the father of the child would have greater success.
  *D. children usually attain bowel control by the age of 30 months.

Reference: p. 1269

Descriptors: 1. 44   2. 03   3. Application
            4. 5 = Implementation 5. Moderate

6. A client with chronic constipation tells the nurse that he would like to improve his diet. Besides encouraging high-fiber foods, the nurse should instruct the client to

  *A. drink 2000 to 3000 mL of fluid daily.
   B. refrain from eating spicy foods.
   C. eat more processed cheese daily.
   D. avoid milk products.

Reference: p. 1270

Descriptors: 1. 44   2. 03   3. Application
            4. 5 = Implementation 5. Moderate

7. The nurse has instructed a client with chronic constipation about high-fiber foods. The nurse determines that the client understands the instructions when he says high fiber in the diet

   A. decreases gas formation when stool is passed.
   B. increases the water reabsorption process.
  *C. serves as a stimulus for peristalsis.
   D. moves the stool more slowly through the intestine.

Reference: p. 1270

Descriptors: 1. 44   2. 03   3. Application
            4. 6 = Evaluation   5. Moderate

8. A client tells the nurse that he has been eating a high-fiber diet for 2 months. The nurse should explain to the client that when the transit time for feces through the colon is decreased, the amount of toxins absorbed is reduced, which can decrease the chance of developing

   A. diverticulitis.
  *B. colon cancer.
   C. constipation.
   D. hemorrhoids.

Reference: p. 1270

Descriptors: 1. 44   2. 03   3. Application
            4. 5 = Implementation 5. Moderate

9. An adult client tells the nurse that she gets diarrhea and feels bloated when she eats ice cream and other dairy products. The nurse determines that the client is most likely experiencing

  *A. lactose intolerance.
   B. diverticulitis.
   C. chronic diarrhea.
   D. gall bladder disease.

Reference: p. 1270

Descriptors: 1. 44   2. 03   3. Application
            4. 3 = Analysis/Diag. 5. Moderate

10. A hospitalized adult client on a regular diet tells the nurse that she has had two episodes of diarrhea. In helping the client to select items from the hospital's menu, the nurse should instruct the client to choose

   A. coleslaw.
  *B. lean meat.
   C. cauliflower.
   D. chocolate brownie.

Reference: p. 1270

Descriptors: 1. 44   2. 03   3. Application
            4. 5 = Implementation 5. Moderate

11. A client visits the clinic with her 10-month-old child and tells the nurse that the child has had bulky stools that appear greasy and are foul-smelling. The nurse should instruct the mother that the child should be evaluated for

   A. biliary disease.
   B. meconium ileus.
  *C. cystic fibrosis.
   D. gallstones.

Reference: p. 1270

Descriptors: 1. 44   2. 03   3. Interpretive
            4. 5 = Implementation 5. Moderate

12. A client tells the nurse that he frequently takes an antacid with aluminum for heartburn. The nurse should assess the client for

   A. increased peristalsis.
   B. irritable bowel sounds.
   C. diarrhea.
  *D. constipation.

Reference: p. 1270

Descriptors: 1. 44   2. 03   3. Application
            4. 2 = Assessment   5. Moderate

13. A client has been given a prescription for antibiotics for 10 days. The nurse should instruct the client that his stool may appear

   A. black.
  *B. greenish-gray.
   C. pinkish-red.
   D. whitish-gray.

Reference: p. 1271

Descriptors: 1. 44   2. 03   3. Application
            4. 5 = Implementation 5. Moderate

14. A pregnant client has been taking iron supplements and tells the nurse that her bowel movements produce dark black-colored stools. The nurse determines that the client is most likely experiencing

   A. intestinal bleeding.
   B. acute obstruction.
   C. biliary blockage.
  *D. normal results from iron salts.

Reference: p. 1271

Descriptors: 1. 44   2. 03   3. Interpretive
              4. 3 = Analysis/Diag.   5. Moderate

15. The nurse is preparing to perform a physical assessment of an adult client's abdomen. The nurse should *first*

   A. palpate the abdomen for nodules.
   B. place the client in an upright position.
  *C. auscultate for bowel sounds.
   D. use percussion in all four quadrants.

Reference: pp. 1272–1273

Descriptors: 1. 44   2. 04   3. Application
              4. 5 = Implementation 5. Moderate

16. While auscultating an adult client's abdomen, the nurse hears abnormally intense and frequent bowel sounds. The nurse determines that the client is experiencing

   A. hypoperistalsis.
   B. hyperresonance.
  *C. borborygmus.
   D. diarrhea.

Reference: p. 1273

Descriptors: 1. 44   2. 04   3. Application
              4. 3 = Analysis/Diag.   5. Moderate

17. While auscultating a 2-day postoperative client's abdomen for 5 minutes, the nurse determines that no bowel sounds are present. The nurse suspects that the client may be experiencing

   A. tympanny.
  *B. paralytic ileus.
   C. hyperresonance.
   D. malabsorption.

Reference: p. 1273

Descriptors: 1. 44   2. 04   3. Application
              4. 3 = Analysis/Diag.   5. Moderate

18. The nurse has instructed an adult client how to obtain a stool specimen. The nurse determines that the client understands the directions when she says,

   A. "I should wait to void until after I obtain the stool specimen."
   B. "It's acceptable to place toilet tissue into the container as it is easily removed."
   C. "I should have my regular bowel movement in the commode then place a specimen in the container."
  *D. "I should void first to avoid contaminating the stool specimen."

Reference: p. 1274

Descriptors: 1. 44   2. 05   3. Application
              4. 6 = Evaluation   5. Moderate

19. A client is diagnosed with a bile obstruction and will need surgical intervention. The nurse should instruct the client that bile obstruction can result in the stool to be the color

  *A. white.
   B. green.
   C. pink.
   D. black.

Reference: p. 1275

Descriptors: 1. 44   2. 05   3. Application
              4. 5 = Implementation 5. Moderate

20. The physician asks the nurse to determine if a 4-year-old hospitalized client has pinworms. To observe for pinworms, the nurse plans to obtain

   A. a sterile specimen container.
   B. two tongue blades.
   C. plastic wrapping material.
  *D. clear cellophane tape.

Reference: p. 1276

Descriptors: 1. 44   2. 05   3. Application
              4. 4 = Planning   5. Moderate

21. The nurse has instructed an adult client how to obtain a stool sample to test for fecal occult blood in his home. The nurse determines that the client needs *further* instructions when the client says,

  *A. "If the color on the slide changes to red, I should report this immediately."
   B. "Multiple specimens are usually collected to verify results."
   C. "The hemoccult slide test requires two drops of developer solution."
   D. "If the color on the slide changes to blue, I should report this immediately."

Reference: p. 1276

Descriptors: 1. 44   2. 05   3. Application
              4. 6 = Evaluation   5. Moderate

22. A client is scheduled for a biopsy while having a proctosigmoidoscopy. The nurse should instruct the client that he will have a procedure which uses

    A. radiopaque dye.
    B. barium solution.
    C. a flexible fiberoptic instrument.
 *D. two rigid instruments.

Reference: p. 1276

Descriptors: 1. 44   2. 05   3. Application
            4. 5 = Implementation 5. Moderate

23. An adult client is scheduled to have a series of diagnostic tests for a bowel disorder. Which of the following should the nurse schedule *first*?

    A. Upper GI series with barium
    B. Lower GI series with barium
    C. Endoscopy
 *D. Fecal occult blood test

Reference: p. 1277

Descriptors: 1. 44   2. 05   3. Application
            4. 5 = Implementation 5. Moderate

24. The nurse has explained the esophagogastroduodenoscopy procedure to an adult client. The nurse determines that the client needs *further* instructions about the procedure when the client says,

    A. "I should empty my bladder before this procedure."
 *B. "It is acceptable to leave my dentures in place during the procedure."
    C. "Before the test, I need to sign a consent form."
    D. "A bitter-tasting local anesthetic may be sprayed in my mouth."

Reference: p. 1278

Descriptors: 1. 44   2. 05   3. Application
         4. 6 = Evaluation   5. Moderate

25. The nurse is preparing an adult client for a colonoscopy the evening before the test. The nurse plans to

 *A. administer a tap water enema as ordered 3 to 4 hours before the test.
    B. encourage the client to eat only soft foods 24 to 48 hours before the test.
    C. tape the client's wedding rings on his finger.
    D. teach the client relaxation techniques as sedatives are infrequently ordered.

Reference: p. 1278

Descriptors: 1. 44   2. 05   3. Application
         4. 4 = Planning   5. Moderate

26. The nurse is caring for an adult client who is scheduled to have an upper GI series and small bowel series. Following instructions about the test, the nurse determines that the client understands the instructions when she says,

    A. "This test will help to diagnose and remove any polyps."
    B. "I should drink only clear liquids on the day before the test."
    C. "A bitter-tasting drink will be given before the test."
 *D. "I should fast and avoid smoking after midnight on the day of the test."

Reference: p. 1280

Descriptors: 1. 44   2. 05   3. Application
         4. 6 = Evaluation   5. Moderate

27. The nurse has instructed an adult client about a barium enema test. The nurse determines that the client needs *further* instructions when the client says,

 *A. "I will need to lie perfectly still on the table during the procedure."
    B. "The barium enema may cause abdominal cramping."
    C. "I will have a cleansing enema before the test."
    D. "I should have only clear liquids the evening before the test."

Reference: p. 1281

Descriptors: 1. 44   2. 05   3. Application
         4. 6 = Evaluation   5. Moderate

28. A 65-year-old client visits the clinic with symptoms of the flu which include nausea, vomiting, and diarrhea. The client tells the nurse she has been unable to tolerate food or fluids for three days. A priority nursing diagnosis for the client is

    A. self-care deficit related to weakness.
    B. body image disturbance related to diarrhea.
    C. self-esteem disturbance related to nausea and vomiting.
 *D. fluid volume deficit related to prolonged diarrhea.

Reference: p. 1282

Descriptors: 1. 44   2. 06   3. Application
         4. 3 = Analysis/Diag. 5. Moderate

29. The nurse visits an adult client who had a colostomy six weeks ago. He tells the nurse that he and his wife haven't had sexual intercourse since his surgery because he has to wear the ostomy bag. A priority nursing diagnosis for this client is

A. self-care deficit related to lack of motivation.
B. self-esteem disturbance related to body image changes.
*C. sexual dysfunction related to perceived change in body image.
D. altered elimination pattern related to colostomy.

Reference: p. 1282

Descriptors: 1. 44   2. 06   3. Application
             4. 3 = Analysis/Diag.   5. Moderate

30. An adult client tells the nurse that she has been experiencing a great amount of flatulence in recent weeks. The nurse should instruct the client to avoid foods such as

A. tomatoes.
B. oranges.
*C. cabbage.
D. peas.

Reference: p. 1284

Descriptors: 1. 44   2. 07   3. Application
             4. 5 = Implementation 5. Moderate

31. The nurse has instructed an adult client with a colostomy about nutrition. The nurse determines that the client needs *further* instructions when he says,

*A. "I should avoid low-fiber foods such as ice cream."
B. "Cauliflower may lead to flatulence."
C. "I shouldn't eat peanuts or popcorn."
D. "If I eat an apple, I should remove the skin first."

Reference: p. 1284

Descriptors: 1. 44   2. 08   3. Application
             4. 6 = Evaluation   5. Moderate

32. The nurse is caring for a 74-year-old client on the first postoperative day following abdominal surgery. To aid the client's bowel elimination, the nurse plans to

A. encourage high-fiber foods.
*B. ambulate the client as soon as possible.
C. obtain an elevated toilet seat.
D. turn the client every 4 hours.

Reference: p. 1284

Descriptors: 1. 44   2. 09   3. Application
             4. 4 = Planning   5. Moderate

33. A client who has been receiving intravenous antibiotics for two days tells the nurse that she is now experiencing diarrhea and asks the nurse to have the doctor order an antidiarrheal medication. The nurse should

A. instruct the client to restrict her fluid intake to 1000 mL.
B. contact the physician for an order for oral Colace.
*C. further assess the client because the antibiotics may be the cause.
D. instruct the client that she may need a different antibiotic medication.

Reference: p. 1288

Descriptors: 1. 44   2. 09   3. Application
             4. 5 = Implementation 5. Moderate

34. An adult client has been given a prescription for paregoric to control acute diarrhea. The nurse plans to advise the client to

A. take the medication for two weeks.
*B. avoid operating heavy equipment while on the medication.
C. take the medication with Kaopectate for the greatest effectiveness.
D. limit fluid intake to a maximum of 1000 mL while taking the medication.

Reference: p. 1288

Descriptors: 1. 44   2. 09   3. Application
             4. 4 = Planning   5. Moderate

35. The nurse is caring for an adult client who is taking Colace to assist with bowel elimination. The nurse should instruct the client to

*A. increase the intake of foods high in fat-soluble vitamins.
B. decrease the intake of high-fiber foods.
C. drink two glasses of Gatorade daily.
D. increase the intake of foods high in calcium.

Reference: p. 1288

Descriptors: 1. 44   2. 09   3. Application
             4. 5 = Implementation 5. Moderate

36. The nurse is caring for an adult client who is scheduled for diagnostic tests which require thorough evacuation of the bowel. Before instructing the client about cleansing enemas, the nurse should assess the client for a history of

A. hemorrhoids.
B. lactose intolerance.
*C. heart failure.
D. gallstones.

Reference: p. 1288

Descriptors: 1. 44   2. 09   3. Application
             4. 2 = Assessment 5. Moderate

37. The nurse has instructed a 60-year-old client with frequent constipation about bulk-forming products such as Metamucil. The nurse determines that the client needs *further* instructions when she says,

A. "It takes about 24 hours for this to work for most people."
B. "This product works by absorbing water and stimulating peristalsis."
*C. "I shouldn't use Metamucil if I have kidney disease."
D. "I need to eat more dairy products, such as milk."

Reference: p. 1288

Descriptors: 1. 44　　2. 09　　3. Application
　　　　　　4. 6 = Evaluation　5. Moderate

38. An 84-year-old client visits the clinic and tells the nurse she has had acute diarrhea for the past four days. The nurse should assess the client for

*A. dehydration.
B. fluid retention.
C. flatulence.
D. hemorrhoids.

Reference: p. 1289

Descriptors: 1. 44　　2. 09　　3. Application
　　　　　　4. 2 = Assessment　5. Moderate

39. The nurse is caring for an adult client on the second postoperative day when the client tells the nurse he is "bloated and has a lot of gas." The nurse should encourage the client to

*A. ambulate in the room and hallway.
B. lie in a supine position after meals.
C. perform thigh and leg exercises daily.
D. ask the physician if an enema is needed.

Reference: p. 1289

Descriptors: 1. 44　　2. 09　　3. Application
　　　　　　4. 5 = Implementation　5. Moderate

40. The physician has ordered a rectal tube for an adult client. The nurse caring for the client plans to

A. obtain a size 8 French tube.
B. leave the tube in place for 45 minutes.
C. ask the client to lie in a supine position after insertion of the tube.
*D. use the tube intermittantly every 2 to 3 hours.

Reference: p. 1288

Descriptors: 1. 44　　2. 09　　3. Application
　　　　　　4. 4 = Planning　5. Moderate

41. The nurse has instructed an adult client about the physician's order for a hypertonic solution enema. The nurse determines that the client understands the instructions when the client says,

A. "I'll feel full as there will be 500 mL of solution administered."
B. "This type of enema may result in water intoxication."
*C. "I will receive about 100 mL of solution during the procedure."
D. "This type of enema may result in potassium retention."

Reference: p. 1290

Descriptors: 1. 44　　2. 09　　3. Application
　　　　　　4. 6 = Evaluation　5. Moderate

42. The nurse is caring for a client in the home who tells the nurse that her stools "look like rock hard marbles." The nurse should contact the client's physician for an order for an enema termed

*A. oil retention.
B. carminative.
C. hypertonic.
D. normal saline.

Reference: p. 1290

Descriptors: 1. 44　　2. 09　　3. Application
　　　　　　4. 5 = Implementation 5. Moderate

43. The nurse is planning to administer an enema to an adult client with chronic obstructive pulmonary disease and rheumatoid arthritis. The nurse plans to place the client in which of the following positions?

A. Fowler's
B. Knee-chest with head of bed elevated
C. Side-lying while flat in bed
*D. Side-lying with head of bed elevated

Reference: p. 1291

Descriptors: 1. 44　　2. 09　　3. Application
　　　　　　4. 4 = Planning　5. Moderate

44. The nurse is preparing to administer an oil retention enema. Following instructions about the procedure, the nurse determines that the client understands the procedure when he says,

*A. "I need to hold the enema for at least 30 minutes if possible."
B. "This enema is being given to help me with my flatus."
C. "The solution will feel cold when the procedure starts."
D. "I shouldn't use this type of enema if I have hemorrhoids."

Reference: pp. 1290, 1291

Descriptors: 1. 44　　2. 09　　3. Application
　　　　　　4. 6 = Evaluation　5. Moderate

45. The nurse prepares to give an adult client a solution of Colyte to cleanse the client's bowels before surgery. The nurse should instruct the client that he will

   A. have a full liquid diet the evening before surgery.
   B. begin having a bowel movement within 30 minutes after consuming the solution.
   C. tolerate the solution more readily if it is warmed to room temperature.
   *D. have a clear liquid diet 24 hours before the administration of the Colyte solution.

   Reference: p. 1291

   Descriptors: 1. 44   2. 07   3. Application
                4. 5 = Implementation 5. Moderate

46. The nurse is caring for a 75-year-old client who tells the nurse that she has not had a bowel movement for three days and is having stool seepage on her bed sheets. The nurse suspects the client is most likely experiencing

   *A. fecal impaction.
   B. hemorrhoids.
   C. constipation.
   D. paralytic ileus.

   Reference: p. 1291

   Descriptors: 1. 44   2. 07   3. Application
                4. 3 = Analysis/Diag. 5. Moderate

47. The nurse is preparing to administer a cleansing enema to an adult client. After donning disposable gloves, the nurse should

   A. elevate the solution to 8 to 10 inches above the client's anus.
   *B. give the solution slowly over a period of 5 to 10 minutes.
   C. position the client on his right side in the Sims' position.
   D. ask the client to hold his breath if cramping occurs.

   Reference: pp. 1292–1293

   Descriptors: 1. 44   2. 07   3. Application
                4. 5 = Implementation 5. Moderate

48. The physician has ordered "enemas until clear" for an 80-year-old client prior to a barium enema. The nurse should instruct the client that

   A. 200 mL of solution will be administered.
   B. the client will be placed on a bedpan.
   *C. no more than three enemas will be administered.
   D. the last enema given should be retained for 30 minutes.

   Reference: p. 1294

   Descriptors: 1. 44   2. 07   3. Application
                4. 5 = Implementation 5. Moderate

49. The nurse has instructed an adult client about rectal suppositories which have been ordered for the client. The nurse determines that the client needs *further* instructions when the client says,

   *A. "I should leave the suppository in place for at least 5 minutes."
   B. "After insertion of the suppository, I should ambulate in the room."
   C. "The suppository will be inserted about 4 inches into my rectum."
   D. "The suppository will be lubricated prior to insertion."

   Reference: p. 1295

   Descriptors: 1. 44   2. 07   3. Application
                4. 6 = Evaluation   5. Moderate

50. The nurse is caring for a client with a temporary colostomy on the second postoperative day. While assessing the client's stoma, the nurse should notify the physician if the stoma color is

   A. pink.
   B. red.
   C. pale.
   *D. purple.

   Reference: p. 1295

   Descriptors: 1. 44   2. 08   3. Application
                4. 3 = Analysis/Diag. 5. Moderate

51. The nurse is caring for a client on the first postoperative day following abdominal surgery which resulted in the client having an ileostomy. The nurse should instruct the client that the drainable ileostomy pouch should

   *A. begin filling within 24 to 48 hours.
   B. begin filling within 72 to 96 hours.
   C. be changed every day.
   D. disposed of once it is half-full.

   Reference: p. 1298

   Descriptors: 1. 44   2. 08   3. Application
                4. 5 = Implementation 5. Moderate

52. The nurse has instructed a client about care of his colostomy. The nurse determines that the client understands the instructions when he says,

   A. "I should plan to drain the pouch when it is completely full."
   B. "I should take only liquid medications if I need them."
   C. "It's important to cleanse around the stoma with alcohol."
   *D. "If I need to go on a trip, I should pack extra pouches and equipment."

   Reference: p. 1302

   Descriptors: 1. 44   2. 08   3. Application
                4. 6 = Evaluation   5. Moderate

53. The enterostomy nurse has instructed an adult client with a permanent colostomy about control of odors. The nurse determines that the client needs *further* instructions when she says she should

*A. avoid milk and dairy products.
B. use bismuth subgallots with meals.
C. eat dark green leafy vegetables daily.
D. avoid foods such as cauliflower.

Reference: p. 1302

Descriptors: 1. 44   2. 08   3. Application
             4. 6 = Evaluation   5. Moderate

54. The nurse is caring for a client who has had diarrhea for the past three days. After instructing the client about care of clients with diarrhea, the nurse determines that the client understands the instructions when he says,

A. "I should avoid hot foods as this can aggravate the problem."
*B. "Cold and spicy foods should be avoided."
C. "It's important to use toilet paper around the anus."
D. "I should continue to take my mineral oil daily."

Reference: p. 1305

Descriptors: 1. 44   2. 09   3. Application
             4. 6 = Evaluation   5. Moderate

55. After 3 days of diarrhea, the nurse determines that the client's diarrhea has subsided when the client has a regularly formed stool. To aid in restoring the client's normal bowel flora, the nurse should encourage the client to consume

A. whole grain products.
B. dark leafy vegetables.
C. skim milk.
*D. yogurt.

Reference: p. 1305

Descriptors: 1. 44   2. 09   3. Application
             4. 5 = Implementation 5. Moderate

CHAPTER 45
Oxygenation

1. In the human body, lungs will become stiff and alveoli will collapse when there is a reduction in

A. cilia.
B. mucous.
*C. surfactant.
D. pleurae.

Reference: p. 1312

Descriptors: 1. 45   2. 01   3. Factual
             4. 1 = No Process   5. Easy

2. In the human body, the stimulus for respiration is

A. positive pressure in the pleural spaces.
B. decreased air pressure in the terminal alveoli.
*C. increased blood carbon dioxide levels.
D. movement of the intercostal muscles.

Reference: pp. 1313, 1315

Descriptors: 1. 45   2. 02   3. Factual
             4. 1 = No Process   5. Easy

3. A client diagnosed with atelectasis will have decreased

*A. diffusion.
B. perfusion.
C. inhalation.
D. friction.

Reference: p. 1314

Descriptors: 1. 45   2. 02   3. Factual
             4. 1 = No Process   5. Easy

4. While assessing a newborn infant, the nurse observes that the infant has an irregular abdominal breathing pattern with a respiratory rate of 50 per minute. The nurse should

*A. continue to monitor the infant.
B. notify the pediatrician.
C. turn the infant to a side-lying position.
D. elevate the head of the crib.

Reference: p. 1316

Descriptors: 1. 45   2. 03   3. Application
             4. 5 = Implementation 5. Moderate

5. While assessing a 78-year-old client, the nurse observes that the client appears to be leaning forward while sitting upright in a chair. The nurse determines that this is most likely due to

*A. kyphosis.
B. senile emphysema.
C. rheumatoid arthritis.
D. barrel chest.

Reference: p. 1316

Descriptors: 1. 45   2. 03   3. Application
             4. 3 = Analysis/Diag.   5. Moderate

6. The nurse is performing a physical assessment on a 12-year-old child. The nurse anticipates that normal findings for the client's breath sounds will be

A. loud with harsh crackles at end of deep inspiration.
B. a harsh expiration longer than inspiration.
*C. clear inspiration longer than expiration.
D. clear inspiration equal to expiration.

Reference: p. 1316

Descriptors: 1. 45   2. 03   3. Application
             4. 2 = Assessment   5. Moderate

7. While assessing breath sounds of a moderately obese client, the nurse would anticipate that the client frequently experiences

    A. asthmatic attacks.
    B. pleural friction rubs.
    C. hypoxic episodes.
    *D. chronic bronchitis.

    Reference: p. 1316

    Descriptors: 1. 45   2. 04   3. Application
              4. 3 = Analysis/Diag.   5. Moderate

8. Before administering morphine intramuscularly to an adult postoperative client, the nurse should assess the client's

    A. pain tolerance.
    B. activity level.
    C. blood pressure.
    *D. respirations.

    Reference: p. 1317

    Descriptors: 1. 45   2. 04   3. Application
              4. 2 = Assessment   5. Moderate

9. While caring for a client with bronchial asthma, the nurse instructs the client that asthmatic attacks have been associated with

    A. morbid obesity.
    *B. generalized anxiety.
    C. decreased fluid intake.
    D. food allergies.

    Reference: p. 1318

    Descriptors: 1. 45   2. 04   3. Application
              4. 5 = Implementation 5. Moderate

10. To assess a client's vocal fremitus the nurse should

    A. percuss the sounds over the fifth intercostal space.
    B. auscultate from the apex to the base of the lungs.
    C. observe movement of the chest walls.
    *D. palpate over a non-bony area of the chest.

    Reference: p. 1319

    Descriptors: 1. 45   2. 05   3. Application
              4. 2 = Assessment   5. Moderate

11. While assessing an adult client, the nurse detects a loud, low booming sound in both lungs. The nurse determines that the client needs further evaluation as this finding most likely indicates

    A. pneumonia.
    *B. emphysema.
    C. tuberculosis.
    D. bronchitis.

    Reference: p. 1319

    Descriptors: 1. 45   2. 05   3. Application
              4. 3 = Analysis/Diag.   5. Moderate

12. The nurse is assessing a client's respiratory system when the nurse detects high pitched sounds at the end of inspiration at the base of the lungs. The nurse should document these sounds as

    *A. fine crackles.
    B. coarse crackles.
    C. wheezes.
    D. rhonchi.

    Reference: p. 1321

    Descriptors: 1. 45   2. 05   3. Application
              4. 3 = Analysis/Diag.   5. Moderate

13. While performing a respiratory assessment of an adolescent client, the nurse detects high-pitched, squeaky sounds on both inspiration and expiration. The nurse determines that the client is most likely experiencing

    A. pneumonia.
    B. bronchitis.
    C. emphysema.
    *D. asthma.

    Reference: p. 1321

    Descriptors: 1. 45   2. 05   3. Application
              4. 3 = Analysis/Diag.   5. Moderate

14. While assessing an adult client's respiratory system, the nurse detects a dry, grating sound while auscultating the lungs. The sound appears on inspiration and is unaffected by the client's coughing. The nurse determines that the client is most likely experiencing

    A. asthma.
    B. chronic bronchitis.
    C. emphysema.
    *D. pleural friction rub.

    Reference: p. 1321

    Descriptors: 1. 45   2. 05   3. Application
              4. 3 = Analysis/Diag.   5. Moderate

15. The nurse has instructed a client about thoracentesis. The nurse determines that the client understands the instructions when she says,

    *A. "Fluid will be aspirated from the plural cavity using a syringe."
    B. "I will probably need to have a general anesthetic."
    C. "I'll be transferred to the operating room for the procedure."
    D. "No more than 500 mL of fluid will be removed."

    Reference: p. 1321

    Descriptors: 1. 45   2. 08   3. Application
              4. 6 = Evaluation   5. Moderate

16. Following a thoracentesis, the nurse should prepare the client for

A. excessive sputum output.
B. intravenous therapy.
*C. chest x-ray.
D. CAT scan.

Reference: p. 1324

Descriptors: 1. 45   2. 08   3. Application
           4. 5 = Implementation 5. Moderate

17. The nurse has instructed an adult client about spirometry testing. The nurse determines that the client needs *further* instructions when the client says,

A. "I should wear the nose clip while breathing through the mouthpiece."
B. "If I take bronchodilator drugs, I should not take them before the test."
*C. "I should wear a tight belt during the procedure."
D. "I may feel very fatigued after the test."

Reference: p. 1322

Descriptors: 1. 45   2. 08   3. Application
           4. 6 = Evaluation   5. Moderate

18. The nurse is preparing an adult client who is to have an arterial blood gas drawn. The nurse should instruct the client that the

A. preferred site is the femoral artery for adult clients.
B. procedure is less uncomfortable than having venous blood drawn.
C. normal pH of the blood is between 7.46 and 7.56.
*D. procedure requires a pressure dressing for 3 minutes after the blood is drawn.

Reference: p. 1322

Descriptors: 1. 45   2. 08   3. Application
           4. 5 = Implementation 5. Moderate

19. An adult client is ordered to have a cytologic study performed on his sputum. The nurse plans to

*A. collect the specimen in the morning before breakfast.
B. collect the specimen in the evening after supper.
C. use the client's saliva if sputum cannot be obtained.
D. ask the client to use a mouthwash after the specimen is collected.

Reference: p. 1323

Descriptors: 1. 45   2. 08   3. Application
           4. 5 = Implementation 5. Moderate

20. An adult client is scheduled for an endoscopy. The nurse should instruct the client that he will most likely have

A. clear liquids the evening before the test.
B. no food or fluids for 4 hours after the test.
C. cold salt-water gargles after the test.
*D. a sedative about 30 minutes before the test.

Reference: p. 1323

Descriptors: 1. 45   2. 08   3. Application
           4. 5 = Implementation 5. Moderate

21. A client has just returned to his hospital room following endoscopy where a biopsy was obtained. The nurse plans to observe the client for

A. hypoxia.
B. nausea.
C. chills.
*D. hemoptysis.

Reference: p. 1324

Descriptors: 1. 45   2. 08   3. Application
           4. 4 = Planning   5. Moderate

22. The nurse has instructed a client about a ventilation detection scan. The nurse determines that the client needs *further* instructions when she says,

A. "I will breathe radioactive gas by mask and then exhale it into room air."
*B. "A radiopaque dye will be injected and then my chest will be scanned."
C. "The radioactive isotope disintegrates in about 8 hours."
D. "This procedure is usually done after the perfusion scan in the x-ray department."

Reference: p. 1324

Descriptors: 1. 45   2. 08   3. Application
           4. 6 = Evaluation   5. Moderate

23. A moderately obese adult client with emphysema tells the nurse that she becomes short of breath after walking one block. A priority nursing diagnosis for the client is

A. ineffective individual coping related to inactivity.
B. fatigue related to overeating and obesity.
*C. activity intolerance related to shortness of breath.
D. fear related to disabling respiratory illness.

Reference: p. 1325

Descriptors: 1. 45   2. 06   3. Application
           4. 3 = Analysis/Diag.   5. Moderate

24. An adult client is receiving morphine every 3 hours for terminal lung cancer and is semi-conscious. A priority nursing diagnosis for this client is

    A. impaired verbal communication related to cancer.
    B. activity intolerance related to pain and medication.
    C. altered oral mucous membranes related to morphine therapy.
    *D. risk for aspiration related to reduced level of consciousness.

    Reference: p. 1325

    Descriptors: 1. 45   2. 06   3. Application
                 4. 3 = Analysis/Diag.   5. Moderate

25. An adult client is ordered to have pulse oximetry with a spring tension sensor. The nurse plans to

    A. cleanse the site with betadine solution and dry thoroughly.
    B. assess the client's pulse at a site farthest from the oximetry sensor.
    *C. remove the sensor every 2 hours and assess skin irritation.
    D. allow the sensor to remain in place continuously.

    Reference: p. 1326

    Descriptors: 1. 45   2. 08   3. Application
                 4. 4 = Planning   5. Moderate

26. The nurse is caring for a client on the first postoperative day following abdominal surgery. The physician has ordered incentive spirometry for the client. The nurse should instruct the client to

    *A. complete the breathing exercises 10 times every hour.
    B. hold his breath and count to 10 before using the spirometer.
    C. breathe through his nose while using the spirometer.
    D. leave any dentures in place during the exercises.

    Reference: p. 1330

    Descriptors: 1. 45   2. 08   3. Application
                 4. 5 = Implementation 5. Moderate

27. A client returns to the hospital unit with a chest tube in place because of a pneumothorax. The nurse should explain to the client that the purpose of the chest tube is to

    A. apply suction to the chest cavity.
    B. provide adequate oxygenation.
    *C. allow the compressed lung to reexpand.
    D. drain fluid from the pleural space.

    Reference: p. 1330

    Descriptors: 1. 45   2. 07   3. Application
                 4. 5 = Implementation 5. Moderate

28. The nurse is caring for a first day postoperative client who has been taught deep breathing and coughing exercises. The nurse plans to

    *A. frequently remind the client to perform these exercises.
    B. instruct the client to cough after meals.
    C. use endotracheal suctioning to stimulate coughing.
    D. encourage the client to cough while in a side-lying position.

    Reference: p. 1331

    Descriptors: 1. 45   2. 08   3. Application
                 4. 5 = Implementation 5. Moderate

29. A client is given a prescription for codeine as a cough suppressant. Following instructions, the nurse determines that the client needs *further* instructions when he says that the medication

    A. can be addictive.
    B. may cause drowsiness.
    C. is a very effective cough suppressant.
    *D. prevents the release of histamine.

    Reference: p. 1331

    Descriptors: 1. 45   2. 07   3. Application
                 4. 6 = Evaluation   5. Moderate

30. A client with very thick, tenacious secretions is given a prescription for an expectorant. Following instructions about the medication, the nurse determines that the client needs *further* instructions when she says,

    A. "I should use a humidifier in my room at night."
    B. "I should drink an adequate amount of fluids."
    *C. "It's acceptable to take an antihistamine with this medicine."
    D. "Robitussin is widely used as an expectorant in cough medicines."

    Reference: p. 1332

    Descriptors: 1. 45   2. 07   3. Application
                 4. 6 = Evaluation   5. Moderate

31. The nurse is caring for an 86-year-old client with unilateral lung disease on her left side. The nurse plans to

    A. alternate the client's position from Fowler's to lying on the left side.
    B. keep the client in high-Fowler's position most of the day.
    C. use oxygen at 2 L by nasal cannula as needed.
    *D. alternate the client's position from semi-Fowler's to lying on the right side.

    Reference: p. 1332

    Descriptors: 1. 45   2. 07   3. Application
                 4. 4 = Planning   5. Moderate

32. An adult client has been ordered percussion to loosen pulmonary secretions. The nurse should

   *A. allow the client to wear a nightgown or underwear during the procedure.
   B. percuss the area below the ribcage then move upward toward the ribs.
   C. percuss the client's lungs over bare skin to better hear the sounds.
   D. continue the procedure even if the client expresses pain.

   Reference: p. 1332

   Descriptors: 1. 45   2. 08   3. Application
                        4. 5 = Implementation 5. Moderate

33. The nurse has instructed a caregiver how to perform postural drainage on her son. The nurse determines that the client needs *further* instructions when the caregiver says,

   A. "I should perform the procedure 1 to 2 hours after meals."
   *B. "I should perform the procedure at least once a day for 1 hour."
   C. "The Trendelenburg position helps drain the lower lobes of the lungs."
   D. "The procedure should be performed 2 to 4 times a day for 20 to 30 minutes."

   Reference: p. 1333

   Descriptors: 1. 45   2. 07   3. Application
                        4. 6 = Evaluation   5. Moderate

34. A client has been prescribed a bronchodilator which is to be administered using a metered-dose inhaler. The nurse should instruct the client to

   A. hold the container upside down before using it.
   B. inhale the medication rapidly through the nose.
   C. exhale after inhaling the medication.
   *D. inhale the medication through the mouth and not the nose.

   Reference: p. 1335

   Descriptors: 1. 45   2. 07   3. Application
                        4. 5 = Implementation 5. Moderate

35. The physician has ordered epinephrine subcutaneously for a dyspneic client. The nurse plans to

   *A. position the client in an upright position.
   B. instruct the client to reduce sodium intake.
   C. observe the client for prolonged bleeding.
   D. monitor the client's blood sugar level.

   Reference: p. 1336

   Descriptors: 1. 45   2. 08   3. Application
                        4. 4 = Planning   5. Moderate

36. An adolescent client is given a prescription for cromolyn sodium (Intal) for asthma. The nurse should instruct the client that the medication

   *A. is useful for prevention of asthmatic attacks.
   B. may cause constipation in clients with lactose intolerance.
   C. may cause changes in blood sugar levels.
   D. can be used to treat acute asthmatic episodes.

   Reference: p. 1336

   Descriptors: 1. 45   2. 07   3. Application
                        4. 5 = Implementation 5. Moderate

37. A client is to be discharged on home oxygen therapy at 2 L/min using a nasal cannula. The nurse plans to instruct the client to

   A. humidify the oxygen with sterile water.
   *B. avoid open flames and smoking.
   C. humidify the oxygen with distilled water.
   D. wear only synthetic fabric clothing.

   Reference: p. 1338

   Descriptors: 1. 45   2. 07   3. Application
                        4. 4 = Planning   5. Moderate

38. A client is to have oxygen therapy at home using a nasal cannula. The nurse should explain that one of the disadvantages of the nasal cannula is that it

   A. requires a tight seal around the nose.
   B. is impractical for long term therapy.
   *C. can easily become dislodged.
   D. makes it difficult to eat or talk.

   Reference: p. 1340

   Descriptors: 1. 45   2. 07   3. Application
                        4. 5 = Implementation 5. Moderate

39. The nurse is caring for a client who is to have a very precise oxygen concentration delivered due to respiratory problems. The nurse plans to obtain a

   A. partial rebreather mask.
   B. nonrebreather mask.
   C. simple mask.
   *D. Venturi mask.

   Reference: p. 1340

   Descriptors: 1. 45   2. 08   3. Application
                        4. 4 = Planning   5. Moderate

40. A hospitalized client is ordered to have continuous oxygen by mask. The nurse plans to

   *A. remove the mask every 2 to 3 hours.
   B. place powder around the mask for greater comfort.
   C. place the mask loosely around the client's nose and mouth.
   D. use cotton balls around the client's ears and scalp.

   Reference: p. 1343

   Descriptors: 1. 45   2. 08   3. Application
                        4. 4 = Planning   5. Moderate

41. The nurse is caring for a 4-year-old client who is receiving oxygen through an oxygen tent. The nurse plans to

   A. open the tent frequently to monitor the client.
   B. keep the tent secured under the client's pillow.
  *C. check the oxygen concentration every 4 hours.
   D. fill the nebulizer with normal saline.

Reference: p. 1345

Descriptors: 1. 45   2. 08   3. Application
                4. 4 = Planning   5. Moderate

42. An adult client is receiving humidified oxygen by mask. The nurse should explain to the client that the purpose of humidifying the oxygen is to

   A. prevent oxygen toxicity.
  *B. prevent drying of the mucous membranes.
   C. decrease the potential for combustion.
   D. provide a route for inhalation medication.

Reference: p. 1345

Descriptors: 1. 45   2. 08   3. Application
                4. 5 = Implementation 5. Moderate

43. The nurse is preparing to insert an oropharyngeal airway into an adult client. The nurse should

   A. rotate the airway 90° as it passes the uvula in the client's mouth.
   B. position the client in a side-lying position before beginning the procedure.
   C. leave dentures in place unless they are broken.
  *D. insert the airway with the curved tip pointing upward toward roof of the mouth.

Reference: p. 1346

Descriptors: 1. 45   2. 08   3. Application
                4. 5 = Implementation 5. Moderate

44. The nurse has instructed a caregiver of an adult client how to care for the client's cuffed tracheostomy tube. The nurse determines that the caregiver needs *further* instructions when the caregiver says,

  *A. "The outer cannula can be removed for cleaning and replaced."
   B. "The tube should be deflated before oral feeding."
   C. "The tracheostomy dressing should be kept dry."
   D. "I shouldn't use cotton balls to clean around the opening."

Reference: pp. 1346–1348

Descriptors: 1. 45   2. 08   3. Application
                4. 6 = Evaluation   5. Moderate

45. The nurse is preparing to perform tracheal suction of a postoperative client who has an endotracheal tube. The nurse should

   A. instill a small amount of normal saline into the airway to liquify secretions.
   B. use a suction catheter of the same size as the endotracheal tube.
   C. wear sterile gown and gloves to perform the suctioning.
  *D. stop suctioning immediately if the client becomes cyanotic.

Reference: p. 1348

Descriptors: 1. 45   2. 08   3. Application
                4. 5 = Implementation 5. Moderate

46. The nurse is preparing to suction an unconsious adult client with an endotracheal tube. The nurse plans to

  *A. use sterile technique for the procedure.
   B. place the client in a supine position.
   C. adjust the wall suction to 10 to 15 mm Hg.
   D. estimate the distance from the client's nose to xyphoid process.

Reference: p. 1349

Descriptors: 1. 45   2. 08   3. Application
                4. 4 = Planning   5. Moderate

47. Following oropharyngeal suctioning of a postoperative client, it is important for the nurse to assess the client's

   A. blood pressure.
   B. apical pulse rate.
   C. nail bed color.
  *D. breath sounds.

Reference: p. 1351

Descriptors: 1. 45   2. 08   3. Application
                4. 2 = Assessment   5. Moderate

48. The nurse is preparing to suction an adult client with a tracheostomy tube in place. The nurse plans to

   A. use aseptic technique.
  *B. hyperoxygenate the client.
   C. place the client in a supine position.
   D. set the portable suction unit at 100 to 120 mm Hg.

Reference: p. 1352

Descriptors: 1. 45   2. 08   3. Application
                4. 4 = Planning   5. Moderate

49. A nurse is caring for a client when the client begins to choke while eating. The client becomes cyanotic and clutches his throat. The nurse should

   A. ask the client if he needs assistance.
   B. administer four thrusts to the client's back.
   C. instruct the client to cough forcefully.
   *D. administer four abdominal thrusts to the client.

   Reference: p. 1357

   Descriptors: 1. 45   2. 08   3. Application
                4. 5 = Implementation 5. Moderate

50. The nurse is planning to clean the nondisposable inner cannula of a client with a tracheostomy. The nurse should obtain

   *A. hydrogen peroxide.
   B. Betadine solution.
   C. sterile water.
   D. distilled water.

   Reference: pp. 1355, 1357

   Descriptors: 1. 45   2. 08   3. Application
                4. 5 = Implementation 5. Moderate

51. The nurse has instructed a group of nursing students how to perform cardiopulmonary resuscitation. The nurse determines that one of the students needs *further* instructions when the student says,

   A. "I should always follow blood and body substance precautions."
   B. "The automated external defibrillator can analyze a person's heart rhythm."
   C. "I should call for assistance before beginning to administer breaths."
   *D. "I should administer four quick breaths, then call for help."

   Reference: p. 1358

   Descriptors: 1. 45   2. 08   3. Application
                4. 6 = Evaluation   5. Moderate

CHAPTER 46
Fluid, Electrolyte, and Acid–Base Balance

1. Plasma is a type of fluid termed

   A. intracellular.
   B. interstitial.
   *C. intravascular.
   D. hypotonic.

   Reference: p. 1367

   Descriptors: 1. 46   2. 02   3. Factual
                4. 1 = No Process   5. Easy

2. Which of the following clients would be more prone to fluid volume deficits due to a greater amount of extracellular fluid? A/an

   A. obese 45-year-old male
   B. obese 50-year-old female
   C. average weight 68-year-old female
   *D. 6-month-old female infant

   Reference pp. 1367–1368

   Descriptors: 1. 46   2. 02   3. Factual
                4. 1 = No Process   5. Easy

3. Which of the following substances would be considered a nonelectrolyte?

   *A. Urea
   B. Sodium
   C. Potassium
   D. Magnesium

   Reference: p. 1368

   Descriptors: 1. 46   2. 02   3. Factual
                4. 1 = No Process   5. Easy

4. The chief electrolyte of extracellular fluid is

   A. potassium.
   B. magnesium.
   C. glucose.
   *D. sodium.

   Reference p. 1369

   Descriptors: 1. 46   2. 02   3. Factual
                4. 1 = No Process   5. Easy

5. A client tells the nurse that he needs to have greater amounts of potassium in his diet. The nurse should suggest that the client eat

   A. nuts.
   B. whole-grain breads.
   *C. bananas.
   D. spinach.

   Reference: p. 1370

   Descriptors: 1. 46   2. 03   3. Application
                4. 5 = Implementation 5. Moderate

6. A solution that has the same concentration of particles as plasma is considered to be

   *A. isotonic.
   B. hypotonic.
   C. hypertonic.
   D. osmolaric.

   Reference: p. 1372

   Descriptors: 1. 46   2. 03   3. Factual
                4. 1 = No Process   5. Easy

7. The type of pressure whereby force is exerted by a fluid against the container wall is termed

A. filtration.
B. oncotic.
C. metabolic.
*D. hydrostatic.

Reference: p. 1373

Descriptors: 1. 46   2. 04   3. Factual
4. 1 = No Process   5. Easy

8. The role of the adrenal glands in maintaining fluid homeostasis is to

A. regulate the conservation of potassium.
*B. regulate the conservation of sodium.
C. increase glomerular filtration.
D. inhibit the release of ADH.

Reference: p. 1374

Descriptors: 1. 46   2. 05   3. Factual
4. 1 = No Process   5. Easy

9. In the body, the parathyroid glands regulate

A. blood volume.
B. sodium.
*C. calcium.
D. extracellular fluid.

Reference: p. 1375

Descriptors: 1. 46   2. 03   3. Factual
4. 1 = No Process   5. Easy

10. If a client is experiencing alkalosis, the client's kidneys will

*A. retain hydrogen ions.
B. retain bicarbonate ions.
C. excrete sodium ions.
D. exrete potassium ions.

Reference p. 1377

Descriptors: 1. 46   2. 06   3. Factual
4. 1 = No Process   5. Easy

11. Fluid intake is primarily regulated by the thirst mechanism. The thirst control center is located within the

A. thalamus.
B. parathyroid.
*C. hypothalamus.
D. pituitary.

Reference: p. 1373

Descriptors: 1. 46   2. 05   3. Application
4. 1 = No Process   5. Easy

12. The nurse is caring for a newly admitted client who has experienced a severe burn as a result of a house fire. The nurse plans to assess the client for

A. weight loss.
B. hypovolemia.
C. hypervolemia.
*D. third-space shift.

Reference: p. 1377

Descriptors: 1. 46   2. 07   3. Application
4. 4 = Planning   5. Moderate

13. The nurse is caring for a client who is in congestive heart failure. The nurse plans to assess the client for

*A. edema.
B. hypovolemia.
C. weight loss.
D. dehydration.

Reference: p. 1377

Descriptors: 1. 46   2. 07   3. Application
4. 4 = Planning   5. Moderate

14. The nurse is caring for a hospitalized adult client following pancreatic surgery. The nurse observes that the client has decreased skin turgor, dry mucous membranes, and a weak radial pulse rate of 120 beats per minute. The nurse determines that the client is most likely experiencing

A. hypervolemia.
B. interstitial to plasma shift.
C. hypernatremia.
*D. hypovolemia.

Reference: p. 1378

Descriptors: 1. 46   2. 07   3. Application
4. 3 = Analysis/Diag.   5. Moderate

15. The nurse is caring for an adult client following abdominal surgery when the nurse observes that the client's urine output is less than 30 mL per hour. The client has an impaired swallowing. The nurse should encourage the client to increase fluid intake by drinking

A. iced tea.
B. hot chocolate.
*C. vanilla milk shake.
D. lemonade.

Reference: p. 1378

Descriptors: 1. 46   2. 07   3. Application
4. 5 = Implementation   5. Moderate

16. The nurse is caring for a client with congestive heart failure who has edema in her hands and feet. Following instructions about decreasing the edema, the nurse determines that the client needs *further* instructions when she says,

  *A. "I should avoid eating bananas until the edema is decreased."
  B. "I should lie down frequently during the day."
  C. "I need to maintain a sodium-restricted diet."
  D. "I should avoid over-the-counter drugs until checking with the physician."

  Reference: p. 1379

  Descriptors: 1. 46   2. 07   3. Application
                4. 6 = Evaluation   5. Moderate

17. The nurse is caring for a client who is at risk for hyperkalemia because of kidney disease. The nurse should notify the client's physician immediately if the nurse observes that the client has

  A. pitting edema.
  B. 2-pound weight loss.
  C. nausea and vomiting.
  *D. an irregular pulse rate.

  Reference pp. 1380, 1382

  Descriptors: 1. 46   2. 07   3. Application
                4. 3 = Analysis/Diag.   5. Moderate

18. The nurse is caring for a client who is taking the diuretic spironolactone. The nurse has instructed the client about the potential for hyperkalemia. Following the instructions, the nurse determines that the client needs *further* instructions when the client says,

  A. "I should use salt substitutes sparingly."
  B. "I should avoid foods such as dried apricots and dried beans."
  *C. "I should avoid regular salt while eating."
  D. "If I develop muscle weakness, I should call my physician."

  Reference: p. 1382

  Descriptors: 1. 46   2. 07   3. Application
                4. 6 = Evaluation   5. Moderate

19. The nurse is caring for a postoperative client following thyroid surgery. The client complains of tingling in her fingers, and muscle cramps. The nurse notifies the client's physician as the client is most likely experiencing

  *A. hypocalcemia.
  B. hypercalcemia.
  C. hypermagnesemia.
  D. hypophosphatemia.

  Reference: p. 1382

  Descriptors: 1. 46   2. 07   3. Application
                4. 3 = Analysis/Diag.   5. Moderate

20. The nurse has instructed a caregiver of a home-bound client with breast cancer about the potential for hypercalcemia. The nurse determines that the caregiver needs *further* instructions when the caregiver says,

  *A. "I should reduce her fluid intake during the day."
  B. "She shouldn't take any antacids for an upset stomach."
  C. "I should call the physician if she demonstrates confusion."
  D. "I should be sure she gets adequate bulk in her diet."

  Reference p. 1383

  Descriptors: 1. 46   2. 07   3. Application
                4. 6 = Evaluation   5. Moderate

21. The nurse is caring for a client who has had diabetic ketoacidosis and has been taking calcium supplements. To determine if the client is experiencing hypomagnesia, the nurse should assess the client for

  A. flushing of the skin.
  B. hypotension.
  C. decreased reflexes.
  *D. tachyarrhythmia.

  Reference: p. 1384

  Descriptors: 1. 46   2. 07   3. Application
                4. 2 = Assessment   5. Moderate

22. While caring for a client with compromised renal function studies, the nurse notes that the client is to receive magnesium citrate in preparation for a lower GI diagnostic test. The nurse should

  A. administer the medication the evening before the test.
  B. observe the client for increased respirations after administration of the medication.
  C. reschedule the lower GI diagnostic test for another date.
  *D. withhold the medication and contact the client's physician.

  Reference p. 1384

  Descriptors: 1. 46   2. 07   3. Application
                4. 5 = Implementation 5. Moderate

23. A client with severe burns is recovering from his injuries and receiving phosphorus in his TPN solution. The nurse should

  A. administer the phosphorous over a 2-minute period.
  B. monitor the client for symptoms of hypercalcemia.
  *C. observe the client for signs of infection.
  D. assess the client for symptoms of constipation.

  Reference: p. 1385

  Descriptors: 1. 46   2. 07   3. Application
                4. 5 = Implementation 5. Moderate

24. The nurse is caring for a 70-year-old client with hyperthyroidism when the client tells the nurse that he uses a Fleet's enema once or twice per week for constipation. The nurse should assess the client for symptoms of

A. hypocalcemia.
B. hypokalemia.
C. hypernatremia.
*D. hyperphosphatemia.

Reference: p. 1385

Descriptors: 1. 46   2. 07   3. Application
              4. 2 = Assessment   5. Moderate

25. The nurse is caring for an adult client with pneumonia who has an arterial blood gas which has a pH of 7.30, a $PaCO_2$ of 48 mm Hg, and a normal HCO_3^-. The nurse determines that the client is experiencing

*A. respiratory acidosis.
B. respiratory alkalosis.
C. metabolis acidosis.
D. metabolic alkalosis.

Reference: p. 1387

Descriptors: 1. 46   2. 07   3. Application
              4. 3 = Analysis/Diag.   5. Moderate

26. A severely anxious client visits the emergency room complaining of lightheadedness and epigastric pain. The client's arterial blood gas reveals a pH of 7.49, $PaCO_2$ of 33 mm Hg, and a HCO_3^- of 21 mEq/L. The nurse determines that the client is most likely experiencing

A. respiratory acidosis.
*B. respiratory alkalosis.
C. metabolic acidosis.
D. metabolis alkalosis.

Reference: p. 1387

Descriptors: 1. 46   2. 07   3. Application
              4. 3 = Analysis/Diag.   5. Moderate

27. The nurse is caring for a postoperative client who has diabetes mellitus. The nurse observes that the client appears drowsy and confused with a respiratory rate of 28 per minute. The client's arterial blood gas reveals a pH of 7.23, a $PaCO_2$ of 33 mm Hg, and an HCO_3^- of 20 mEq/L. The nurse notifies the client's physician of the arterial blood gas results because the client is most likely experiencing

*A. metabolic acidosis.
B. metabolic alkalosis.
C. respiratory acidosis.
D. respiratory alkalosis.

Reference: pp. 1388, 1390

Descriptors: 1. 46   2. 07   3. Application
              4. 3 = Analysis/Diag.   5. Moderate

28. The nurse is caring for an adult client who has gastric suction following surgery. The client tells the nurse that he has tingling in his fingers and is feeling dizzy. The client's arterial blood gas reveals a pH of 7.50, a $PaCO_2$ of 48 mm Hg, and HCO_3^- of 27 mEq/L. The nurse notifies the client's physician as the client is most likely experiencing

A. metabolic acidosis.
*B. metabolic alkalosis.
C. respiratory acidosis.
D. respiratory alkalosis.

Reference: p. 1388

Descriptors: 1. 46   2. 07   3. Application
              4. 3 = Analysis/Diag.   5. Moderate

29. The nurse is assessing a client's fluid, electrolyte, and acid–base balance. During the nursing admission interview, an appropriate question for the nurse to ask to gain subjective data from the client is

A. "Have you had any recent vomiting?"
B. "Do you take any medications, such as aspirin?"
*C. "Describe the type of fluid intake and amounts during the last 24 hours."
D. "Describe how much you perspire in a 24 hour period."

Reference: p. 1390

Descriptors: 1. 46   2. 08   3. Application
              4. 5 = Implementation 5. Moderate

30. During an admission interview with the nurse, the client tells the nurse that he has experienced a "lot of edema in the past few days." The best response by the nurse is to ask the client

A. if he adheres to a low-sodium diet.
B. if he has had any recent laboratory blood studies.
C. when he last had a physical examination.
*D. what interventions have been attempted with results.

Reference: p. 1390

Descriptors: 1. 46   2. 07   3. Application
              4. 5 = Implementation 5. Moderate

31. The nurse is caring for an adult client with numerous draining wounds from gunshots. The nurse should assess the client for

A. third-space shifting.
B. intracellular fluid deficit.
*C. extracellular fluid deficit.
D. metabolic alkalosis.

Reference: p. 1390

Descriptors: 1. 46   2. 08   3. Application
              4. 2 = Assessment   5. Moderate

126

32. The nurse plans to weigh a client daily to determine the client's fluid balance status. The nurse plans to weigh the client

   *A. before breakfast.
   B. after breakfast.
   C. after supper.
   D. before bedtime.

   Reference: p. 1391

   Descriptors: 1. 46   2. 08   3. Application
                4. 4 = Planning   5. Moderate

33. The nurse is caring for an adult client with hypovolemia and malnutrition. While performing a urine specific gravity on the client's urine, the nurse anticipates that the specific gravity will be

   A. 1.001 to 1.010.
   B. 1.015 to 1.020.
   *C. 1.025 to 1.030.
   D. 1. 040 to 1.050.

   Reference: p. 1391

   Descriptors: 1. 46   2. 08   3. Application
                4. 3 = Analysis/Diag.   5. Moderate

34. A 4-year-old client is admitted to the hospital with hypovolemia. To test the client's skin turgor, the nurse should pinch the client's skin over the

   A. sternum.
   B. forearm.
   C. ankle.
   *D. abdomen.

   Reference: p. 1393

   Descriptors: 1. 46   2. 08   3. Application
                4. 5 = Implementation   5. Moderate

35. While caring for a 6-year-old child, the nurse observes that the client has difficulty salivating. The nurse contacts the child's physician as the nurse determines that the client is most likely experiencing

   A. metabolic acidosis.
   *B. fluid volume deficit.
   C. fluid volume excess.
   D. sodium excess.

   Reference: p. 1393

   Descriptors: 1. 46   2. 08   3. Application
                4. 3 = Analysis/Diag.   5. Moderate

36. The nurse is caring for a client with congestive heart failure when the client asks the nurse, "Why are my hands so swollen?" The nurse should explain to the client that the edema is due to retention of

   *A. sodium.
   B. potassium.
   C. magnesium.
   D. phosphorous.

   Reference: p. 1394

   Descriptors: 1. 46   2. 07   3. Application
                4. 5 = Implementation   5. Moderate

37. The nurse is preparing to assess the vital signs of a client with hypovolemia following surgery. The nurse anticipates that the client's pulse will be

   A. slow.
   *B. rapid.
   C. irregular.
   D. normal.

   Reference: p. 1394

   Descriptors: 1. 46   2. 08   3. Application
                4. 2 = Assessment   5. Moderate

38. The nurse assesses an adult client who is hospitalized for pneumonia. While assessing the client's breath sounds, the nurse detects fine, moist crackles. The nurse determines that the client is experiencing

   A. hyponatremia.
   B. hypercalcemia.
   *C. fluid volume excess.
   D. fluid volume deficit.

   Reference: p. 1395

   Descriptors: 1. 46   2. 08   3. Application
                4. 3 = Analysis/Diag.   5. Moderate

39. While assessing an adult client's blood pressure, the nurse determines that the blood pressure is 120/82 in the supine position and 100/76 while in the sitting position. The nurse determines that the client is most likely experiencing

   A. third-space shifting.
   B. increased extracellular fluid.
   C. hypomagnesemia.
   *D. fluid volume deficit.

   Reference: p. 1395

   Descriptors: 1. 46   2. 08   3. Application
                4. 3 = Analysis/Diag.   5. Moderate

40. The nurse is planning to test for Chvostek's sign on an adult client. The nurse should

   A. use a rubber percussion hammer over the client's knee.
   *B. percuss the facial nerve about 2 cm anterior to the earlobe.
   C. use a blood pressure cuff and inflate above systolic pressure for 1 minute.
   D. visualize the external jugular veins on both sides of the neck.

   Reference: p. 1395

   Descriptors: 1. 46   2. 08   3. Application
                4. 5 = Implementation   5. Moderate

41. The nurse is preparing to test for Trousseau's sign in an adult client. Before the assessment, the nurse instructs the client that the test requires the nurse to

   A. percuss the client's deep tendon reflexes using a rubber hammer.
   B. auscultate breath sounds to determine if crackles are present.
  *C. use a blood pressure cuff on the arm to inflate the cuff for 3 minutes.
   D. use a penlight to assess the client's jugular veins on both sides of the neck.

Reference: p. 1395

Descriptors: 1. 46   2. 08   3. Application
           4. 2 = Assessment   5. Moderate

42. While caring for an adult client, the client's arterial blood gas reveals that the pH is 7.40, the $PaCO_2$ is 46, and the HCO_3^- is 24. The nurse determines that the client's compensation is

  *A. absent.
   B. partial.
   C. ineffective.
   D. complete.

Reference: p. 1306

Descriptors: 1. 46   2. 08   3. Application
           4. 3 = Analysis/Diag.   5. Difficult

43. The nurse is caring for a client who tells the nurse that he is a highway engineer and must supervise construction and repairs regardless of the weather temperatures. A priority nursing diagnosis for the client is

   A. risk for heat stroke related to occupation and excessive heat.
   B. potential for fluid and electrolyte imbalance related to occupation.
   C. altered urinary elimination related to fluid imbalances.
  *D. risk for fluid volume deficit related to insufficient fluid intake.

Reference: pp. 1396, 1398

Descriptors: 1. 46   2. 07   3. Application
           4. 3 = Analysis/Diag.   5. Moderate

44. The nurse is caring for an 80-year-old client who has congestive heart failure. A priority nursing diagnosis for the client is

   A. risk for injury related to the client's age.
  *B. impaired skin integrity related to edema.
   C. altered cardiac output related to congestive heart failure.
   D. risk for fluid volume deficit related to the client's age.

Reference: p. 1397

Descriptors: 1. 46   2. 07   3. Application
           4. 3 = Analysis/Diag.   5. Moderate

45. An adult client diagnosed with hypovolemia and intravenous therapy needs to have at least 3000 mL of fluid daily; however, her intake has only been 2000 mL during the last 24 hours. An appropriate nursing goal for this client is that the client will

   A. increase her fluid intake by selecting juices that she enjoys.
   B. have a pitcher of ice water at her bedside at all times.
   C. inform the nursing staff when she is thirsty.
  *D. drink an 8-ounce glass of fluid every hour while awake.

Reference: pp. 1397, 1400

Descriptors: 1. 46   2. 09   3. Application
           4. 4 = Planning   5. Moderate

46. The nurse has instructed a caregiver of an 82-year-old client with fluid volume deficit. Following the instructions, the nurse determines that the caregiver understands the instructions when the caregiver says,

   A. "My mother should have at least 3500 mL of fluid daily."
   B. "If I notice that she has edema of her hands, I should increase her potassium intake."
  *C. "If my mother has persistent nausea and vomiting, I should call the physician."
   D. "I should withhold her diuretic medication if she isn't drinking enough fluids."

Reference: p. 1399

Descriptors: 1. 46   2. 09   3. Application
           4. 6 = Evaluation   5. Moderate

47. The nurse is caring for a client with renal disease who is on restricted fluids. The nurse should plan to

   A. offer small amounts of fluid with meals.
   B. use large cups to administer small amounts of fluid.
  *C. serve the client ice chips from time to time.
   D. offer the client hard candy throughout the day.

Reference: p. 1401

Descriptors: 1. 46   2. 09   3. Application
           4. 4 = Planning   5. Moderate

48. To avoid the potential for a fatality, the nurse should use extreme caution when injecting a client with

   A. sodium.
   B. calcium.
   C. magnesium.
  *D. potassium.

Reference: p. 1402

Descriptors: 1. 46   2. 09   3. Application
           4. 5 = Implementation 5. Moderate

49. A homebound client is receiving intravenous therapy through a Groshong central venous catheter with a transparent dressing. When making a home visit to the client, the nurse should assess the client for

*A. symptoms of infection.
B. hypoglycemia.
C. nausea and vomiting.
D. urinary retention.

Reference: p. 1403

Descriptors: 1. 46   2. 09   3. Application
              4. 2 = Assessment   5. Moderate

50. The nurse is caring for a client who will be receiving IV antibiotics through a peripherally inserted central catheter (PICC). Following instructions about the PICC, the nurse determines that the client needs *further* instructions when she says,

*A. "I can expect to have more pain with this type of catheter."
B. "This type of catheter is less costly than other types."
C. "This type of IV access has a decreased risk of pneumothorax."
D. "Multiple venipunctures are unnecessary with this type of catheter."

Reference: p. 1404

Descriptors: 1. 46   2. 09   3. Application
              4. 6 = Evaluation   5. Moderate

51. The nurse is preparing to start an intravenous infusion on an adult client. The nurse plans to

A. place the tourniquet 2 inches above the selected site.
B. place an ice pack over the intended vein for greater access.
*C. use a circular motion to cleanse from the center of the site outward.
D. don sterile gloves before inserting the intravenous catheter.

Reference: p. 1406

Descriptors: 1. 46   2. 09   3. Application
              4. 5 = Implementation   5. Moderate

52. The nurse is caring for a client who is to have an implanted port central venous catheter inserted. The nurse should instruct the client that the catheter will be placed into which vein?

A. Basalic
B. Antecubital
C. Cephalic
*D. Subclavian

Reference: p. 1409

Descriptors: 1. 46   2. 09   3. Application
              4. 5 = Implementation   5. Moderate

53. A client is ordered to have 1000 mL of D_5W infused over a 10-hour period. The solution set delivers 60 gtt per mL. The number of drops per minute that should be administered by the nurse is

A. 25.
B. 50.
*C. 100.
D. 125.

Reference: p. 1413

Descriptors: 1. 46   2. 09   3. Application
              4. 5 = Implementation   5. Moderate

54. The nurse is caring for a client who has been receiving intravenous therapy for 48 hours when the nurse observes that the site of the intravenous catheter is cool and swollen. The nurse plans to

A. notify the client's physician.
B. continue to monitor the client's IV site.
C. flush the tubing with normal saline.
*D. discontinue the IV and restart it at another site.

Reference: pp. 1419–1420, 1422

Descriptors: 1. 46   2. 09   3. Application
              4. 5 = Implementation   5. Moderate

55. The nurse is caring for a client who has been receiving intravenous fluids and intravenous antibiotics for 72 hours. When the nurse observes the client's blood pressure is elevated and there is neck vein distention, the nurse notifies the physician as the client is most likely experiencing

A. an allergic reaction to the antibiotics.
*B. fluid overload.
C. speed shock.
D. pulmonary embolism.

Reference: p. 1422

Descriptors: 1. 46   2. 09   3. Application
              4. 3 = Analysis/Diag.   5. Moderate

56. The nurse is caring for a client who is to have a blood transfusion. The nurse should plan to

A. use a #21 size catheter to start the intravenous therapy.
B. assess the client's blood pressure every 5 minutes during the first half hour.
C. initiate an intravenous infusion of D_5W solution.
*D. ask the client if he has ever had a reaction to blood in the past.

Reference: pp. 1425, 1428

Descriptors: 1. 46   2. 10   3. Application
              4. 4 = Planning   5. Moderate

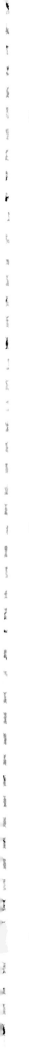